Trevor

Believe in

You!

Go all in boddy.

James.

IRON COWBOY

REDEFINE IMPOSSIBLE.
50 IRONMAN TRIATHLONS, 50 STATES, 50 DAYS.

BY
JAMES LAWRENCE

IN MEMORY OF TIM WATSON

Tim:

A friend and brother whose life was cut short. Thanks for the laughs, the memories, and some incredible journeys! Thank you for encouraging excellence, particularly in your family and closest friends, through always giving 100% no matter what activity we were competing in. Your desire to always win pushed us to work harder and be better. We miss your quick-witted trash talk, your competitive spirit, and your contagious smile. Thanks for all the laughs, the memories and for sharing your incredible life's journey with us.

We miss you!

TABLE OF CONTENTS

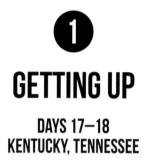

GETTING UP

DAYS 17–18
KENTUCKY, TENNESSEE

I was woken by the tickle of lips against my beard and by the sound of those same, familiar lips whispering in my ear.

"James."

When I opened my eyes, I saw my wife, Sunny, seated beside me on the fold-out bed I'd passed out on fifteen minutes earlier while sipping kombucha during a break between the cycling and running segments of today's solo triathlon. The only other people inside the motor home were my wingmen, Casey and Aaron, workhorses responsible for everything from preparing my morning oatmeal to driving me through the night to the next state. They stood looking down on me gravely from the foot of the bed.

"You have to get up, love," Sunny said gently. "It's almost seven. You need to start running."

I have to get up.

This simple thought released in me the mother of all sinking feelings. A gory blister in the nail bed of the second toe of my left foot that had been bothering me since Missouri had become increasingly painful during the last hour of the ride I'd just completed. When I got off my bike and put my full weight on the foot, it felt as if I had been shot by a staple gun.

To complete today's triathlon, I now had to run a full marathon, a task requiring approximately 15,000 high-impact landings on each foot—or 15,000 more staple shots. In the best-case scenario, the torture would last until one o'clock a.m. In the worst case, it would end much earlier, when I couldn't take the pain anymore and quit, abandoning my dream that was years in the making. My next triathlon was scheduled to start 300 miles and one time zone away (we'd lose an hour en route), in Chattanooga, at six o'clock a.m.

Sunny slipped an arm behind my back and raised me to a sitting position. I buried my hands in my face and began to tremble. More than one hundred local supporters were waiting for me with audible restlessness outside the motor home. I had not slept longer than five hours in eighteen nights.

"I can't do this anymore!" I sobbed. "I just can't!"

Sunny rubbed my back in slow circles, saying nothing more until I'd cried myself out. We both knew I wasn't really giving up. I just couldn't hide my suffering behind a brave face any longer; I needed to let it out, to be vulnerable, and to ask for help.

"Come on, let's get you changed," Sunny said. "I'll run with you. If you can't run, we'll walk. We will do it together."

I nodded.

Aaron hustled to hand me the bin that contained my running gear for the day. I stripped off my wet cycling shorts and put on a pair of knee-length black running shorts with American flag side stripes, clean socks, a headband, and running shoes. Then we filed out of the motor home and into a steamy, southern summer evening. A smattering of cheers and applause greeted my appearance, and I mustered a bleak smile in response.

Everyone was wearing the Iron Cowboy 5K race numbers that our eldest and youngest children, Lucy (twelve) and Quinn (five), had distributed while their dad was procrastinating, napping, and weeping in private. These two were now palling around with the middle three—Lily (eleven), Daisy (nine), and Dolly (seven)—and some of the many kids who had come out with their parents from their homes here in Henderson, Kentucky, and from across the bridge in Evansville, Indiana. Out of school for the summer, Sunny's and my blond brood had spent the day at an Airbnb house, the day's ninety-nine-degree heat, with unbearable humidity, having spoiled their plans to visit an amusement park.

The 5K had been both the shrewdest and most naïve idea we'd come up with in planning this campaign, the Fifty, as we called it. Inviting all comers to run the final 3.1 miles of each triathlon's marathon leg had proven to be an effective way to get local communities involved in our mission. The presumption that I would never fail to complete all but the last 3.1 miles of each triathlon by the advertised 5K start time

❶ GETTING UP

of seven o'clock had been laughably optimistic.

By Day 6 in Nevada, we were already behind schedule and losing would-be participants who weren't interested in waiting until after dark for the privilege of running with me. It took us three more days to implement the obvious solution of starting the 5K at seven o'clock no matter how far I had managed to run by that time. Now here I was on Day 17 having failed to complete a single step of the marathon before seven.

Before each 5K, I delivered a short speech. Today's participants formed a half-circle around me, smiling expectantly.

"I'm James Lawrence, also known as the Iron Cowboy," I began.

On any other day, I would have gone on to thank my local supporters and talk about my goal of drawing attention to the problem of childhood obesity. Unfortunately, today my heart just wasn't in it because of my suffering.

"My toes are messed up," I said instead. "I'm just going to walk. Don't bother waiting for me."

With this rousing battle cry, the Iron Cowboy 5K began. The herd stampeded away from me as I limped along behind them with Aaron, Sunny, Lucy (making good on a pledge to do all fifty 5Ks with me), and my seldom-seen project manager, Jordan. The first landing of my left foot brought an involuntary grimace to my face, but I kept going in the hope that the mysterious analgesic effect of exercise would kick in and dull the discomfort. It did not. After two blocks, I'd had about all I could take. I stopped.

"This isn't going to work," I said. "We need to think of something."

The five of us brainstormed together and came up with the plan of finding a pharmacy and scoring some lidocaine. With any luck, it would numb the pain just enough to allow me to finish. We resumed walking south through Atkinson Park toward the center of town. Fifth Street looked promising, so we turned there. But within two blocks the pain forced me to stop for a second time.

"I need to lance this sucker," I said to Sunny.

"Do you want me to run back and grab your cuticle clippers?" Sunny asked.

I sat down on a strip of grass by the sidewalk and removed my left shoe and sock. Sunny was back in a few minutes. I gently poked the instrument between the toenail and cuticle, poised to snip. I might as well have stabbed myself with a red-hot kebab skewer. My foot recoiled like a startled animal. I handed the clippers back to Sunny with a disappointed shake of my head.

Just then, a young man dressed to run approached us. Eric, as he introduced himself, had arrived at the park just after the 5K began and had dashed after the crowd in the hope of catching up with me. Eyes focused on his target, he had run right by me without knowing it and had circled back after learning I was struggling.

"I heard you've got some blisters," Eric said.

"You heard correctly," I said.

Eric removed a running pack from his back and pulled out moleskin, duct tape, and superglue.

"You brought all that for a 5K?" I asked.

"I was planning to run with you longer," Eric said, blushing. "Is there anything here you can use?"

"What we need is a pharmacy," Sunny said. "We're hoping a little lidocaine might give him some relief. Is there a drugstore around here?"

Eric worked his cell phone and discovered there was a Rite Aid two blocks away. He ran off, having insisted on paying for the medication himself. We followed behind at a walk. When Eric exited the store, bag in hand, he found me circling the parking lot, inching painfully toward accumulating 26.2 miles of GPS-measured distance on my Garmin watch (it didn't matter where or how slowly I did so, only *that* I did). I plopped down on the curb, bared my hideous foot again, and applied the medication.

It did nothing. A block away from the store, I was once again sitting on a patch of grass and contemplating my mutinous toe. Just then a couple came along, also dressed in running clothes. I recognized the male half of the pair, Tom, as one of my earlier cycling companions. (Anyone was welcome to join me for any amount of swimming, biking, or running during the day.)

"This is my wife, Kelly," he said. "She's a physician."

"Really? You're a doctor?" I asked, a bit too incredulously. Sunny later teased me for thinking Kelly was too young and pretty to be an MD.

"Yes, I'm a doctor," Kelly said, narrowing her eyes at her husband. "But I'm afraid I can't help you with your feet; I don't have any supplies with me."

"I don't care," I said. "Just tell me what to do with it."

Kelly crouched down and inspected the toe. She shook her head. "This stuff you've wrapped it with is worthless," she said. Tom suggested toe caps that he used but told us that they would have to be ordered. He promised to order some for us right away, and ship them to an address in a future state. Tom and Kelly agreed to later meet us at a pizza joint, where my supporters would be gathering after completing the 5K, in an effort to wrap my toes as best as she could, to try to relieve some pain. Jordan and Aaron went there directly while Sunny and I returned to the motorhome to fetch a different pair of shoes, in an attempt to relieve my toes. Rockhouse Pizza is located inside an old gray-brick building on a quiet corner in downtown Henderson. At the threshold, I paused my watch. I had covered only 4.63 miles of my marathon. It was already eight thirty. The restaurant was packed with runners. At a corner table, I spied five blond children. *My* family! Casey had gathered them up and brought them there in hopes of lifting my spirits, and it worked. They squealed with delight because they each got to order a glass of soda! They had smiles on their faces as they enjoyed their pizza and the buzz of the restaurant. For a moment my toe was forgotten.

Also present were Aaron, Jordan, and his wife, Jessa, the campaign's official photographer. No sooner had we joined them than we were approached by the owner of the establishment, Dave, a triathlete himself and another member of the day's cycling group. He offered us anything we wanted on the house. I ordered a large pizza with pepperoni, ham, bacon, sausage, beef, green peppers, mushrooms, onions, black olives, tomatoes, and banana peppers. It arrived quickly, and I destroyed five slices even quicker.

I had started the Fifty intending to maintain the same clean, natural diet that I followed back home, which I had developed over several years with input from my wife, my coach, David, and my chiropractor, Dallas. That intention had gone straight out the window when I ran smack into the reality of needing 10,000 to 12,000 calories a day to survive.

Tom and Kelly wandered in and found our table. For the fourth time in an hour, I took off my shoe and sock. "That's probably not a very appetizing sight," Tom said, frowning at my bad toe and gesturing toward the other eaters.

"These are my people!" I laughed. "Just wrap it!"

Twenty-six minutes after I sat down (according to my watch), I stood up again, having decided to try to finish the marathon back at the park. I would be able to do a quarter-mile loop, choosing whether I walked or ran. My official Kentucky host (or "ambassador," in the lexicon of the Fifty), Jim, left the restaurant with us and stationed himself under a pop-up tent beside the path, fishing cold drinks out of an ice chest for me whenever I got thirsty, which was often. An older guy named Neil came along also, and Dave followed along half an hour later. The kids played outside while

Sunny, concerned about time, tried various ways of hustling me along. She suggested I try running the long sides of the oval and walking the short sides. I obediently broke into a herky-jerky trot, but after ten or twelve excruciating steps, I gave up.

"Okay, how about we run the short sides and walk the long ones?"

I looked at my wife, and she knew there was no way I was running. Even walking was barely tolerable. The kids soon joined me. A couple at a time would do a lap with me. They would walk some with me, then split off and climb on the statues and benches that were on the path. Next thing I knew, they were chasing each other on the grass, and their giggles filled the dark night. I was so grateful that they were so happy, but I struggled not to let my pain consume me.

When it was time for the kids to go to bed (all five slept on the full-sized pullout bed in the middle of the RV or in two twin beds in the back of the RV), I stopped long enough to kiss each of them on top of the head. They begged to stay up until I finished, but we insisted they at least get ready for bed. Sunny gathered them all into the motorhome, as Lucy vowed to stay up until I finished. She wanted to see me after I had completed the day, to make sure that I was okay. Jim excused himself at eleven thirty, saying he had to go to work at four.

That left three of us. Dave, Neil, and I shuffled along together under a crescent moon, talking sporadically. Neil told me he had recently lost more than fifty pounds and that he had never run or walked farther than ten miles before today. The mention of distance prompted Dave to ask me how far we had to go.

"I don't want to know," I said firmly.

It was approaching two o'clock in the morning when I looked at my watch and saw the number I wanted to see: 26.20 miles.

"Where can I get cleaned up?" I asked my escorts.

The motorhome had a shower, but it was cramped and only had cold water. I used it only as a last resort.

"I live half a mile from here," Neil said. "You can shower there."

When we got to Neil's place, I was dismayed to discover he lived in a second-floor apartment. I walked backward up the stairs. While I scrubbed the stink off my body, Neil blended smoothies for us. He said they had been a key contributor to his weight loss. This made me smile, thinking of my sweet wife who insisted that I drink a smoothie every day. I couldn't count how many very green smoothies that I had consumed in preparation for this adventure.

It was pushing three o'clock when Neil dropped me off at the park. Upon returning to the motorhome, Lucy had fought to stay awake, but was sleeping peacefully with the rest of my family. I looked around, felt the silence, and thought of my love and appreciation for my family. I strapped on my NormaTec compression boots, which would squeeze my sore muscles while I slept, bringing circulation to them and accelerating the recovery process. I lay down on the pull-out bed that had been the scene of my earlier meltdown. Sariah, who worked for one of my sponsors, ZYTO, and whose primary job was to use a high-tech ZYTO scanner to assess my nutritional needs, jabbed an IV needle into my arm. I'd been taking saline infusions as needed since Day 8 in New Mexico when an emergency saline IV had brought me back from the brink of total physical collapse. I was unconscious long before the saline bag had emptied.

Just before he took the wheel to begin the long drive to Chattanooga, Casey snapped the long day's last photo to post on Facebook. The positioning of my body in the bed made it appear as though I were lying in a coffin. My body at that point bore more than a passing resemblance to a corpse.

A sudden awareness of falling ripped my eyelids open. I was on my bike, veering off the road to the right. Reflexively, I threw my weight in the opposite direction. Now I was falling in *that* direction. I landed hard on my left side and skidded briefly. A man's voice called out from behind, "Stay down! Don't move!"

A man came over, dressed in cycling clothes, and kneeled down next to me. A small crowd of other cyclists gathered around us. The man asked me a number of questions and examined various parts of my body. He seemed to know what he was doing. Convinced that I hadn't broken my neck, he sat me up. A police cruiser with flashing lights was parked on the shoulder of the road just ahead, and an officer was walking toward me.

"What am I doing here?" I asked him.

"You mean you don't know?" he said.

"Um, not really."

The policeman told me I was in Chattanooga, Tennessee, and had apparently fallen asleep on my bike. He then walked back to his car and returned promptly with a first-aid kit, which he handed to the man who'd told me to stay down, who then expertly cleaned and dressed abrasions on my hand, elbow, and hip. The hip hurt the most.

A woman asked for my cell phone. As I handed it over, her name popped into my head: Robyn. She'd been with me all day, beginning with a swim in the Tennessee River. Things were starting to come back to me. Robyn called the wingmen and told them what had happened; the wingmen then called Sunny. I could tell from listening to Robyn's side of the conversation that she'd expected them to react hysterically and was both relieved and somewhat disturbed by their nonchalance. Robyn handed the phone back to me and then passed me a small bottle. "Drink that," she said. The label identified the product as an energy shot. I trusted Robyn, but at that moment anyone could have told me to drink anything, and I would have willingly submitted.

"I have to get up," I said, as much to myself as anyone else.

The longer I remained on the ground, the more my body would stiffen, making it harder to get going again. The guy who had told me to stay down, whose name (and occupation) I also now remembered—Doug, fireman—helped me up with a handclasp and an arm pull. I showed off my dressings for some photos to be posted online and then we set off again. My watch showed I had ridden a little more than thirty miles when I went down. I still had eighty-two miles to go—and then another marathon.

My next challenge was finding a position I could ride in comfortably. When I rested my forearms on the time-trial bars, the pain in my banged-up, left forearm intensified. If I moved my hands to the top bar, the worst of my discomfort migrated to my bandaged palm. My hip hurt regardless, and my bad toe was still sore, though not quite as painful as it had been yesterday in Kentucky.

Every now and again, as I coasted down a hill, I tested the mangled digit by lifting it and pressing the blistered nail bed against the top of the shoe, then curling it down into the sole. Even when I wasn't engaging in such masochism, the toe was tender enough that I could feel my pulse in it. If I'd been so inclined, I could have measured my heart rate by looking at my watch and counting the toe throbs.

The police car trailed behind us, lights still flashing, as we pedaled along a tree-lined country road in rising heat. The tunnel vision, caused by severe sleep deprivation, that had precipitated my unconscious tumble did not return. Doug tried to keep me engaged in constant conversation, though it hadn't worked the first time. He'd been doing the same thing before the crash, having become concerned by one or two things I had said that struck him as a little off.

❶ GETTING UP

"Like what?" I asked him.

"Like asking my name three times," he said.

It was seven thirty in the evening and still ninety-three degrees when we returned to our staging area (or home base) at Southern Adventist University. At least sixty people were there waiting to start the Iron Cowboy 5K. I made them wait a little longer while a local massage therapist, Crystal, did what little she could to work out my kinks inside the RV. Sunny soaked the tip of a running sock in Young Living essential oils and handed it to me to put on.

"Are you sure about this? I asked.

In my experience, wet socks *caused* blisters; they did not cure them.

"Trust me," Sunny said confidently.

We ran the 5K on a pristine greenway, 1.55 miles out, 1.55 miles back. I was at the limit of my pain tolerance from the very first stride. Each landing of my left foot sent shock waves up my leg and into the bruised hip socket, triggering an echo of the original crash impact. On the bright side, the pain in my toe seemed minor by comparison.

On the inbound portion of the 5K, a boy on a bike came flying by us from behind on the grass verge. He was passing right next to me when a culvert caught his front tire and launched him into a spectacular accidental flying dismount. The boy's father happened to be running with me. He and another guy, Paul, stopped to help. When I was speaking with Paul later, he told me that when the boy found out that the Iron Cowboy had crashed earlier, had gotten up and kept going, he too got up and kept going.

At the staging area, I hung around for a while in front of the motor home, meeting people, posing for photos, and autographing whatever was handed to me. Rick, my ambassador, stayed close, acting as a handler of sorts.

"I know you're having a rough day," he said in a quiet moment. "You need to come back to Chattanooga when you can actually enjoy this place."

"Oh, I'm fine," I said. "I'm having a good day."

What I meant was that my earlier accident had left me feeling oddly relieved. I had known for some time that a wreck was inevitable—I'd fallen asleep on my bike in previous states. The only question was whether I would get back up when it did happen, and I had.

Night fell and people left. I went inside the motor home to eat and put off completing the marathon. A fan, who happened to be a chiropractor, gave me an adjustment; she was thwarted by my inability to lie on my painful, left side. At 9:45, I sent Casey out to ask my lingering supporters if there was a lighted area nearby where I could run on a soft surface. Paul said he knew just the place. He made a couple of phone calls and got the lights turned on at the Ooltewah High School track.

Another absurdly optimistic assumption we'd made in planning the Fifty was that I would always travel in the motorhome with my family. But the motorhome was slow and needed more time to get from state to state than our smaller vehicles. Sometimes I finished triathlons so late that Sunny was forced to leave me behind to follow along later in the van or the Subaru. Tonight would be one of those nights.

Lieutenant Starnes—the police officer who had tailed me while I was on my bike—drove me to the high school and dropped me off. When Aaron arrived in the Subaru fifteen minutes later, I was already running. The track had been resurfaced two years before and had a nice, rubbery give underfoot. About a dozen supporters had come over from the campus to run with me.

On our first lap, I made a courtesy announcement. "I apologize, but I fart a lot, and I pee a lot," I said. "Now that I've gotten that out of the way, I won't say any more about it."

If nothing else, the Fifty had taught me to do what needed to be done in the most efficient way possible, regardless of social norms. In the days ahead, I wouldn't even bother warning people about my bodily functions.

At midnight it was still eighty-four degrees. My shirtless torso was soaked in sweat. One by one, people said goodbye, wished me luck and drove away. But we gained a body when Lieutenant Starnes returned, having traded his uniform for running clothes. The five or six others remaining with me had already shared their stories. Starnes now shared his.

"Seven years ago," he began, "I weighed 425 pounds."

His daughter, Jessie Anne, was then nine. One day, out of the blue, she told him, "Dad, I want you to get healthier." It was a troublesome thing for Starnes to hear, but he knew that *he had plenty of time, being that he was only forty-four.* Six weeks later, Jessie Anne suffered a brain aneurysm and died. To honor her memory, her father took up exercise, changed his diet, and lost weight—172 pounds.

When the inaugural Ironman Chattanooga took place in September 2014, Starnes decided he would do the race the following year. He became a triathlete, and it was through some of his new training buddies that he heard about the Iron Cowboy and the Fifty, Fifty, Fifty. My cause of fighting childhood obesity struck a chord with him, so when he found out that I was coming to Chattanooga, he got permission from the Hamilton County Sheriff's Office to escort me through my bike ride.

"How far do you have to go?" Paul asked me after Starnes had finished telling his story.

"I don't want to know," I growled.

Around a quarter past one, Paul left to get a couple of hours of sleep before he went to work. But half an hour later he was back with a cooler full of iced towels for my hip, a bag of peanut butter and honey sandwiches, and a jar of honey in case I wanted more.

I grabbed a sandwich, pried the two pieces of bread apart, and gestured toward the jar with my chin. "Load it up," I said. I ate the small sandwich in five or six bites and then ate two more, also with extra honey.

With about three miles left to run, I asked the survivors if they knew of a way I could get into the university's wellness center to take an ice bath, something Robyn had suggested I do after my crash. Lieutenant Starnes told me he would take care of it and departed. I finished the marathon with six others, exchanged damp hugs with them, and hung out for a few more pictures. Aaron had been sleeping in the Subaru out in the parking lot. I knocked on the driver's side window, and he woke up as casually as if he'd only been feigning sleep.

At the entrance to Hulsey Wellness Center, a security guard nodded, swung the door wide, and waved us in. Starnes kept me company while I soaked and Aaron searched the neighborhood for food.

"How the heck do you do this every day?" Starnes asked me.

I heard this question often, and the question puzzled me. People seemed to want to hear something novel, some single nugget of wisdom, that I alone had discovered. The truth was simple; I believed that it was always possible to take one more step. I had this philosophy before the Fifty, and it remained my philosophy eighteen days into the Fifty.

"I don't know," I answered. "I get up. They escort me out the door. I don't want to go, but I know the other part of me does want to go. I get in the water, and I just start swimming."

Aaron came back with a couple of premade sandwiches he'd found at a gas station. One ham, one turkey. Both looked a week old.

"It's all I could find," he apologized.

I opened the ham sandwich and took a bite, chewed, swallowed. It *tasted* a week old. I forced down one more bite and tossed the rest away.

We left the wellness center a few minutes before three in the morning. Aaron and I thanked Starnes and the security guard and shambled over to the Subaru. I climbed in through the hatchback door and sprawled onto a pallet of blankets and sheets. There was only one position I could sleep in given the cramped space and the state of my left hip, and that was a fetal curl on my right side. If my blistered toe so much as touched the hatchback door, as it did a few times over the next six hours, it felt as though a wasp had stung it.

I felt the car speeding up, slowing down, turning one way, turning the other way. Without even opening my eyes I could feel the sun was up. We had to be close. Minutes later, the car stopped, and the engine went silent. The hatchback opened, Aaron looked in at me, and I looked out at him. My neck and my right shoulder were stiff and ached from having been stuck too long in the wrong position. My mouth felt cotton-filled. I had gone to sleep dehydrated and was waking up even more dehydrated. My tongue hurt.

I have to get up.

With no small effort, I propped myself up on my elbow. Aaron seemed very far away, almost unreachable. I wasn't yet thinking about the 2.4 miles of swimming, 112 miles of pedaling, and 26.2 miles of running that lay ahead of me. I was thinking, *How the heck am I going to get out of this car?*

People often ask me what the hardest part of doing fifty iron-distance triathlons, in fifty consecutive days, one in each state, was. The hardest part, honestly, was waking up and getting started.

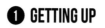 GETTING UP

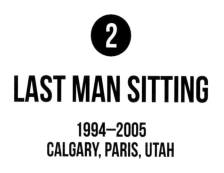

LAST MAN SITTING

1994–2005
CALGARY, PARIS, UTAH

I've always been a dreamer. The big dream of my adolescent years was representing my native Canada at the Olympics in wrestling. This ambition wasn't farfetched, as I went undefeated at 134 pounds in my senior year at William Aberhart High School in Calgary and won the 1994 Alberta provincial championship. The next step in my march toward the Summer Games in Athens was to test my abilities against other top grapplers at the national club championships, held that year in Saskatoon.

I won my opening match easily and then edged out a tough opponent in round two. But when the referee lifted my left arm to signal my second victory, my shoulder exploded in pain. I had torn the middle deltoid muscle during the bout. I never wrestled again.

I was raised Mormon, and in the months leading up to the injury I'd been on the fence about whether to serve a two-year mission abroad, something all members of our church are encouraged to do after high school. My whole life I had been the type of person who followed his heart. I did what felt right and true to my better self and avoided what didn't. But I struggled with this decision.

On the one hand, I sensed strong social pressure to go abroad. A young man who wants to marry a Mormon girl someday, as I did, has a lot more options if he has completed a mission. On the other hand, missionary work would entail approaching strangers in public and talk to them about religion. As an introvert, I didn't think I was cut out for that. But maybe that was just what I needed at that point in my life—to get outside my comfort zone and do something that challenged me to grow in new ways. The abrupt ending of my wrestling career settled it. I put in my papers with the church.

On December 5, 1995, I started two months of intensive missionary training in Provo, Utah, still wearing the sling with which I was outfitted after shoulder surgery. I spent twenty-four hours a day with eleven other apprentices learning French (I would be sent to Paris upon completing my training), brushing up on the gospel, and sleeping in a dormitory. Bonds form quickly in such circumstances, and I became pretty tight with a fellow apprentice named Tim, also a former wrestler. I was disappointed to learn that Tim would serve his mission in Switzerland. Having him with me in Paris for moral support might have made a difference. Then again, probably not.

I lasted six weeks. France is known as one of the toughest places to do a mission. I heard stories of missionaries who returned home after two years there without having baptized a single person. That's a lot of rejection, and I couldn't handle it. I left my apartment each morning queasy with fear. I forgot every last word of French that I knew, even though I had been through bilingual school, as soon as I mustered the gumption to waylay some busy atheist in a park. I flushed with embarrassment each time the inevitable rebuff was uttered. After the worst forty days of my life, I called the mission president and told him I wanted to go home.

I took the next flight to Calgary and moved back in with my parents. My older sisters, Kari and Christine, were already out on their own making successes of their lives. Only the baby, Sandra, seven years my junior, was still at home. I paid $400 a month to live with my parent's, being that I wasn't in school.

As soon as I was settled, I reconnected with my best friend, Quinn. He was the yin to my yang, complementing my quietness with his charisma, my moodiness with his jollity, and even my whiteness with his mixed African and European ancestry. Quinn had cultivated an appealing post-high school lifestyle during my absence. Four nights a week he tended bar at the Fox and Firkin, a popular nightclub. On his nights off he hit the casinos to play blackjack, and by day he golfed at McCall Lake Golf Course, where he held a second job as a caddy.

This lifestyle soon became mine as well. Quinn began to sneak me into McCall, where I embarked on the long process of mastering the game of golf. At first, I hated it because I couldn't put the ball in the hole to save my life. I found that I liked it, the more and more that I improved. Eventually, I found in the genteel pastime a surprisingly fulfilling outlet for my competitive instincts, which had been dammed up since I'd given up wrestling.

I got set up at the Fox and Firkin too, starting as a busboy and eventually advancing to a bartender. It amused Quinn to no end that I had never had a sip of alcohol in my life, I never intended to, being that it was against my religion. For that matter, so was blackjack, yet somehow my faith didn't stop me from becoming rather good at the game under Quinn's tutelage.

I worked four nights a week from four o'clock in the afternoon until two-thirty or three in the morning. From eight o'clock on, the club was a madhouse, with two floors meeting the fire code limit, a line around the block, and three bars serving drinks as fast as we could pour them. After closing, Quinn and I and the other young staffers would go out for breakfast. I'd sleep till noon and golf until my next shift started. Life was good. I was twenty years old, making $1,500 a week, and not tied down to anything. I bought a motorcycle. I got tattoos.

But then all of a sudden I was twenty-three years old, still living at home, and not having *quite* as much fun playing all of the time. A lot of my friends had college degrees now. Kari and Christine had gotten married and started real careers, and I knew my father wanted me to do the same. He never said anything about it—in fact, he barely spoke to me at all—but I knew.

The dreamer in me was still alive but in deep hibernation. The nearest thing to a substitute for the Olympics I could come up with during this period was a lame series of get-rich-quick schemes that I never pursued beyond the first step because my heart wasn't in them.

In June 1999, feeling compelled to adopt a more straight-and-narrow lifestyle and lacking a new dream to save me from the grim path of respectability, I quit the nightclub and took a job as an oil patch worker. The rig I was to work on was located in a remote oil field in northern Alberta. I was given its coordinates—it had no address—and told to find it with a map.

I never did. On the day I was supposed to start my new vocation, I set out from my parents' house in their Mercury Villager minivan and drove in circles for hours until I was just about out of gas, seeing nothing more oil rig–like than barren tundra stretching forever in every direction.

On the way back to Calgary, more relieved than disappointed, I listened to Power 107 ("Today's Best Music") and heard a promotional message that grabbed my attention. The radio station was sponsoring a contest they called the Midway

Marathon. Ten lucky participants would be challenged to ride a Ferris wheel for ten days, from the opening to the closing of the Calgary Stampede, the world's largest rodeo. Any survivors would split a prize of $10,000. I knew two things instantly: one, I *had* to get on that Ferris wheel; and two, if I did, I would win.

The voice on the radio said nine out of the ten slots had already been filled. I had one chance. Listeners were instructed to call in when a particular song (I don't recall which) played, and the seventh caller would get the last seat.

I listened to Power 107 nonstop for the next two days. In the meantime, I took a sales job at a country club, and it was there that I heard the designated song. I seized the nearest phone and dialed the radio station's number as fast as my right index finger would move. When the call was answered, my hopes soared, only to be dashed in the next instant. I was caller number eight. Eight!

But something in me refused to hang up the phone and move on with my life. I begged the producer to take down my name and number and to allow me in as an alternate if any of the ten contestants dropped out. A day before the Calgary Stampede opened, I got the call. Someone had bailed and I was in the big show.

Immediately I phoned my new boss at the country club, Collin.

"I need ten days off," I told him.

"You're fired," he said.

On the morning of July 9, I rode my motorcycle to the fairgrounds and made my way to the Roundup Center. A handful of Power 107 staff was there to receive the contestants. We signed waivers and were given a verbal briefing and a written handout with numbered rules. The contest would start at eight o'clock, with five participants in one car and five in a different car at the opposite side of the wheel. The other cars would remain open to regular public use.

Except for two ten-minute breaks separated by six hours, we would ride non-stop until the wheel shut down at midnight. At that time, we would get a half-hour of free time on the ground and then return to our cars to sleep on the wheel as it sat stationary overnight. At 7:30 in the morning, we would get another thirty minutes on terra firma before the ride started again. Every other night we would be allowed to go home, to bathe and sleep in our own beds.

We could not eat, drink, read, or listen to Walkmans while on the Ferris wheel. All clothing and accessories had to be worn as the manufacturer intended. For example, sunglasses had to remain over the eyes. (I'm not sure what sort of unfair advantage this restriction was intended to prevent, but I wasn't going to question it, much less defy it.) Each car would have a walkie-talkie, and we were instructed to use it to notify the judges when we wanted to quit. If one car lost occupants more quickly than the other, surviving contestants would be redistributed to restore balance.

The contest began. I spent the early rotations checking out the four rivals sharing my cart, a job that was made easier by its circular seating arrangement. A wide range of personalities was represented. We had one chatterbox who got on everyone's nerves quickly. In future years, the Midway Marathon would include a *Survivor* element, with contestants voting one person off the wheel at the end of each day. This dude would have been the first to go. At the opposite end of the dispositional spectrum was an Indian woman who sat stone-faced behind chunky sunglasses and never opened her mouth. She worried me the most.

After five minutes, the ride stopped, and the regular riders got off, and a fresh batch got on. Then the ride started again.

It took less than an hour for the first contestant to snap. I couldn't believe it. Just sitting there was the easiest thing I had ever done. I knew already I would last the full ten days.

When our first break came, I hustled to the nearest restroom to pee. I took a quick glance at myself in a mirror and was alarmed to see I had the beginnings of a nasty sunburn. I would have to remember to ask my parents to bring sunscreen when I saw them later in the day. A rushed walk back to the Ferris wheel left me with six minutes to eat some of the food my mom had packed in Tupperware for me.

Four more contestants quit before midnight. Meanwhile, I was actually enjoying myself. At the top of each rotation, I had a bird's-eye view of the entire rodeo grounds. I made a little game of trying to pick the cute girls out of the crowds of fairgoers below. The southeast corner of the racetrack was just visible from the wheel's twelve o'clock position. When the timing was right, I got a glimpse of horses or chuck wagons speeding through the turn, and what I couldn't see, I could hear: cattle roping, bronco riding, everything.

After dark, things got fun. I had the best seat in the house for the nightly fireworks show. And though I couldn't see Shania Twain performing live on the main stage, her country-pop stylings reached my ears just fine. Midnight arrived surprisingly quickly.

Only one more contestant gave up in the next six days. Those who were susceptible to boredom were weeded out quickly, leaving behind only the types of people who could drive alone cross-country in a car with a broken radio and get all the stimulation they needed from the landscape and their thoughts. The contest was physically challenging to some degree, but not very. I got hot sometimes, cold other times, thirsty, hungry, bladder-full, and stiff from trying to sleep upright on a hard plastic seat. When I went home on the second night and closed my eyes for a moment in the shower, I nearly fell over, feeling my body still moving in a giant vertical loop. But none of these discomforts tempted me to quit.

On the seventh night, a thunderstorm rolled in, with jagged flashes of light and the crackling sounds growing louder and louder. I saw the judges conferring on the ground beneath me, and then a call came over the walkie-talkie. The ride would be suspended until the danger had passed. My three fellow survivors and I were ushered to the edge of the Ferris wheel platform, just far enough from the metal structure to avoid getting zapped, and told to sit still and do nothing. It hardly constituted a reprieve from the monotony of the ride itself. When we were herded back into our cars ninety minutes later, I was thankful.

Day ten started out cold and wet. I suited up in heavy rain gear. As the morning progressed, though, the rain stopped, and the temperature climbed. I became uncomfortably warm, but remembering the contest rules, I resisted the impulse to take off my rain hat or poncho. At the three o'clock and nine o'clock positions of each rotation, I was able to peek into my last rival's car. At one such moment, I thought I noticed something. I waited until the wheel had made another half rotation and looked again.

Sure enough, one of my opponents had dropped the suspenders of his rain pants. *All clothing and accessories must be worn as the manufacturer intended.* I snatched the walkie-talkie and tattled to the judges, who told me they would check into the matter. The next time my opponent's car came around to the bottom, the wheel was stopped. After a brief exchange, he was pulled off the ride, purple-faced and gesticulating wildly.

It was over. I had won. At midnight, I stepped off the wheel for the last time and was handed one of those oversized Publishers Clearing House–style checks, photographed, and interviewed on live radio.

Ten days later, I hitched a ride to Utah to hang out with my friend Tim, from missionary training, and to contemplate my next move. I never went home.

❷ LAST MAN SITTING

In Canada, Thanksgiving is celebrated on a Monday in October. When I woke up on Thursday, November 25, 2004, I was fully accustomed to the American version of the holiday. A lot had changed in five years. I was now married to Sunny, raising two young daughters (Lucy and Lily), and managing the golf department at a sporting goods store in Provo. All these changes were ones I had sought out. But the next big change in my life would come to me unexpectedly, today, and would start me down a new path that would eventually revive the dreamer inside me and reveal the quest I had been born to pursue.

Earlier in the week, Sunny had suggested the two of us run the Orem Turkey Trot—a four-mile Thanksgiving-themed running race—before we took the family over to her parents' place for dinner. Sunny ran every day, and we had bonded initially through exercise. Having met in a psychology class at Utah Valley University, we had our first date at a fitness club. But I was not a runner. I played golf six days a week and lifted weights several days a week when I was really on a roll. Now, twenty-eight, I still saw myself as a high-level athlete, but I had sunk much farther than I recognized, and I had a reality check coming.

Raised with the metric system, I was still getting used to miles, but I figured four miles couldn't be that far. The race started and finished at the Orem Fitness Center, the event's title sponsor. At eight o'clock on Thanksgiving morning, Sunny and I found ourselves mushed together with a few hundred other souls behind the start line. Sunny was content to hang near the back, but sizing up the competition, I felt I should be up front, ahead of the flabby middle-aged guys and the mothers pushing baby joggers.

The horn sounded, and everyone took off. As a first-timer, I didn't know that 80 percent of race participants lose their minds at the start of each race and sprint like kamikazes toward certain disaster, so I made the same mistake. Sunny, who *did* know better, let me go. I hit the one-mile mark after six and a half minutes, and I was in agony. I couldn't believe that my windpipe felt scraped raw by sucked-in air. My heart was an angry fist trying to punch its way out of my chest. My poor legs were so weak that they felt diseased. My pace slowed and then slowed some more. The homestretch was a humiliation, with people I would have sworn could never beat me in any athletic competition passing me by the dozens, including flabby middle-aged guys and mothers pushing baby joggers.

I spent the rest of the day at my in-laws' in a deflated stupor, coughing like a smoker and whining about chest pains. Sunny, meanwhile, was her usual gregarious self. At one point, she fixed me with a look of exaggerated disappointment and said two words I will never forget: "You're pathetic."

As husband and wife, Sunny and I were well-matched in much the same way, Quinn and I were well-matched as friends. Laid-back and jokey, I liked to think I kept my wife from taking herself too seriously. Feisty and no-nonsense, she kept me from not taking myself seriously enough.

Two weeks later, Sunny informed me that she had registered both of us for the Salt Lake City Marathon, then four months away. It was her way of challenging me to overcome being pathetic. To her surprise, I embraced the challenge—albeit in a laid-back way.

Having no idea how to prepare for a marathon, I poked around online and found a minimalist training plan that required only three runs per week. Like many golfers, I tended to think expensive equipment could make up for lack of ability, so I bought the costliest pair of running shoes sold at Copeland's Sports, where I then worked.

As expensive as they were, these shoes did not spare me from developing a bad case of iliotibial band syndrome—pain just above and outside the right knee—that forced me to shut down my training three weeks before race day. The longest run that we had completed to that point was sixteen miles.

On the morning of the marathon, I swallowed half a Lortab—the first pain pill, prescription or otherwise, I'd ever taken (not for religious reasons but rather because I have a personal distaste for medicines of all kinds). Despite my inadequate preparation, I felt more excited than anxious as I stood with Sunny and my friend Mike, with whom I had done all my training, in the start corral, listening to the national anthem of my adopted nation. I looked at the 26.2 miles ahead as a slam-dunk opportunity to redeem my Thanksgiving Day disgrace. The horn sounded, and 80 percent of the people around me again lost their minds, but this time I held back. A little more than eight minutes into the race, feeling great, I heard electronic chirps all around me—GPS watches notifying their wearers they had completed the first mile. *These people are weird,* I thought.

At five miles, I still felt great. What I did not understand at the time was that *everyone* feels great with twenty-one miles left in a marathon, even those who are in way over their heads.

At sixteen miles my body seemed suddenly to remember it had never gone any farther before. My injured knee started to hurt, and soon everything hurt, but I would gladly have chosen the pain over the fatigue. I felt as though my blood were being slowly siphoned out of me. The misery of the last three miles of the marathon made the last three miles of the Orem Turkey Trot seem like a Swedish massage by comparison. I did not see how I could possibly survive to the finish line.

But I did, because no matter how extreme my suffering became, *it was only suffering*. The pain and fatigue I felt made me *want* to stop, but I recognized at every step that I didn't *have* to stop. So I took one more step and asked myself again: *Can I take one more?*

Small steps add up. I completed the marathon in 4:15:31, in 1,140th place, exactly two hours behind the winner. Ten feet beyond the line, I threw up violently, creating a puddle that seemed far too large to have issued from one man's stomach.

We stopped for lunch on the way home from the marathon. Sunny said to Mike and me, "I am NEVER doing that again!" Mike and I both felt the exact same way. I had no intention of ever doing another race, yet in completing this one marathon, I had learned I possessed a certain gift, a gift for endurance. I would have never guessed that the same mental ability that had carried me to victory on the Ferris wheel back in 1999 would help me survive the Salt Lake City Marathon six years later, despite a woeful lack of physical readiness. It was clear to me, quitting was a choice, not a necessity.

In choosing redemption over comfort, I discovered that endurance, whether it entails sitting still and fighting boredom for days on end or running farther in one day than most people drive their cars, is all in the mind.

That same night, Mike and I attended a mixed martial arts event at the E Center in Salt Lake City, having bought tickets several days earlier under the assumption the marathon wouldn't take too much out of us. As it turned out, we both felt as though we'd been hurled out of a moving train, and my injured knee, in particular, was an inferno of hurt. Sitting down was a relief initially, but as the fight card progressed, I felt my legs stiffening. Mike and I were seated at the end of a row, so people were constantly shimmying past us to get food and drinks, forcing me repeatedly to half-stand to make room for their passing. Each time I performed this simple action, it was more challenging and painful. By the start of the main event, which featured Steven "Razor" Sharp and his trademark pink hair, my right knee had swollen to the size of a cantaloupe.

The fight ended, and everyone rose and began to press toward the exits. But when I tried to do the same, I couldn't move. My right leg was now completely locked and unable to bear weight.

"I can't get up!" I told Mike in horrified disbelief.

Not moving very well himself, Mike helped me stand on my left leg. There were two ways out of the building: we could either go up the steps or down the steps to reach an exit. Everyone else in our row had gone up, which was quicker. I gave it a try, but it was a no-go, even with an arm over Mike's shoulder. So we turned around and put gravity to work for us. Our progress was torturously slow, and the building had long since emptied of other fight fans when we reached the landing.

Seeing our plight, one usher sent another usher to fetch me a wheelchair. When it arrived, I stared at it for a long moment, thinking I would almost rather die than be carried helplessly out of the same building I had walked into a few hours earlier after having just run 26.2 miles. But I had no choice. I sat down, Mike grabbed the handles and pushed me out to his car.

The next day at church, the women were sharing good news moments in their class. Sunny spoke up, "Yesterday James and I ran our first marathon." There were cheers and applause, "James was faster than me, but today I can walk and he can't!" Laughter erupted in the group of women, and Sunny laughed even harder. It's not every day that she has an edge on me, so she enjoys it when she gets her moment. After church she approached me as I laid on the couch, still trying to recover well enough to walk, and we laughed together as she reminded me of how great she felt, while I was still suffering.

I knew that the day before we had all sworn off racing ever again, but I felt something gathering inside me. That something was a burning need for a whole new level of redemption, an all-consuming desire not to let this shameful moment define me in any lasting way.

I wanted to race again, as soon as possible.

❷ LAST MAN SITTING

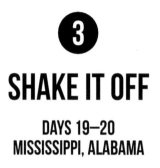

3

SHAKE IT OFF

DAYS 19–20
MISSISSIPPI, ALABAMA

I could tell by the looks I saw on the faces of the handful of Mississippians awaiting my very late arrival at the Courthouse Racquet & Fitness Club that they did not expect the Iron Cowboy to roll into Jackson squished in the rear of a Subaru Outback. Their expressions changed from curious, to puzzled, to disturbed as I dragged myself out of the hatch and hobbled zombielike toward the motor home, which Casey, Sunny, and our children had arrived in a couple of hours earlier.

I disappeared inside and plopped down at the kitchen table. In Chattanooga, the day before, Sunny and the kids had intended to visit the headquarters of McKee Foods, makers of Little Debbie Snack Cakes and other sinful confections. The company didn't offer tours, so an employee arrived with boxes of product for everyone to enjoy. Needless to say, the Wingmen took ownership of these treats and enjoyed them late into the night, as they drove from state to state.

Still half asleep, I was munching on a snack cake and reached for another when a bowl of oatmeal was placed in front of me.

"How's the hip?" Casey asked.

"Not good," I said. "I should probably have it looked at."

Casey went outside and asked my Mississippi ambassador Darryl if there was a doctor in the vicinity. Moments later my wingman returned with Jen, a pediatrician, and triathlete, who had been among those waiting to swim with me. Without standing up, I hitched a thumb over the waistband of my shorts and exposed the wound—now a green-brown bruise raked with glistening red scratches. Jen inspected it briefly.

"It's looking pretty boggy," she said. The medical slang was not familiar to me, but I looked it up later and learned it refers to a sponginess of texture caused by fluid buildup. "Lucky thing you decided not to swim in the reservoir. It might have gotten infected."

Driving into Mississippi, Sunny and Casey discussed concerns regarding the weather warnings that they saw on the billboards heading into town. "Extreme Weather Warning, Plan Accordingly." "What are they talking about?" Casey said to Sunny. She responded, "I don't know, it looks gorgeous. They must know something that we don't know." Sunny looked up the local weather, showing a storm coming in later, while Casey called Kyle, my friend who was doing a lot of coordinating work for the Fifty from his home in Utah. Kyle contacted Darryl right away to see if changes needed to be made. Darryl mentioned the weather warning, and for safety reasons, we moved Day 19 indoors. After taking a lot of heat online from haters, earlier in the campaign, for doing a couple of indoor triathlons to escape a tropical storm, I disliked the idea of going back inside, but I felt I had no choice. It seemed as if this tropical storm was following us.

Jen asked what I'd been using to treat the wound, and Sunny confidently showed her our Young Living Essential Oils.

"That's probably not the best thing," she said. Sunny ignored her and continued treating my wounds with sheer confidence.

After a battle and an excruciatingly long time, my morning swim was finished, and I was back inside the motor home. I was now surrounded by a fresh batch of medical professionals, whom Darryl had rounded up to help me recover from vicious leg cramps, that had forced me to flail across the pool with one working limb—my right arm having been rendered pretty much useless by a shoulder injury suffered on Day 3 in Washington. Trey, a fireman, and his friend Chris, a paramedic, administered an IV, while Helen, a massage therapist, worked on my calves. Karen, a nurse practitioner, soon joined these three.

"What's the problem?" Karen asked.

I had so many problems to choose from that the question threw me momentarily. After mulling it over, I decided to go with the toe. Karen leaned in to take a look at the ghastly mess the second toe of my left foot had become.

"Oh, my gosh!" she said, flinching. "How are you even walking?"

"Actually, it doesn't hurt as much as it did a couple of days ago," I said.

❸ SHAKE IT OFF

"Of course it doesn't," Karen said. "The nerves are dead." She took a second look at the mangled digit. "You've got to take the pressure off that nail bed," she advised. "Every time you land on it, you're cutting off the circulation. That could lead to gangrene."

I waved away this last remark, as I do all bad news from doctors. Faith moves mountains.

"How do I take the pressure off?" I asked.

Karen recommended I cut a section out of the toe area of my left running shoe. She continued her inspection of the roadkill, my toe.

"It's badly infected," she said. "And it looks like the infection is traveling up your lower leg. You should go to the emergency room right away. There's a hospital a quarter mile from here. If you continue, you're going to lose that toe. Maybe the whole foot."

"You know what?" I asked, smiling. "I don't care! That toe has given me nothing but trouble. I say we just cut it off."

This was my way of telling Karen I didn't believe her. She looked at me in horror. Aaron made it worse by laughing. At her wits' end, Karen pulled out her phone and called a wound specialist she knew. I was amused by the obvious difficulty she had in making him understand who her patient was and what he was doing to himself.

"He says he won't come," Karen said after hanging up.

"Why not?" I asked.

"Because if he does come, you won't do what he says."

"Smart guy," I said.

Karen and I finally came to a compromise. I promised to visit the ER after I finished my bike ride, time permitting, and Karen, a triathlete herself, said she would ride with me if only to hold me to my promise. She was just leaving to change into cycling clothes when I thought of something else I needed to ask her.

"Hold on a second," I said. "My mouth really hurts, and I can't taste anything I eat."

I hadn't bothered to mention this to anyone until now. Karen shook her head in exasperation.

"Stick out your tongue," she said.

I did so. Aaron screwed up his face in disgust. I was informed that the organ was blood red and covered with a white film.

"Have you been eating a lot of fruit?" Karen asked.

"Truckloads," I said.

"It's the fruit," she said. "You need to stop eating it for a while. In the meantime, I can prescribe a special mouthwash that should help with the pain." I used this mouthwash for a solid ten days, and it never ended up helping.

Soon after Karen left, I fell asleep. I was still asleep two hours later when Sunny came back to the motorhome with Dolly, whom she'd taken to the dentist. It was after one o'clock in the afternoon.

"How far into the bike is he?" she asked Trey who was there with the IV bag.

"Um, he hasn't started the bike yet ma'am," Trey says fearfully.

Sunny about hit the ceiling, but she knew that she needed to keep her cool. She started to nudge me, and glared at the wingmen who had allowed me to sleep this long.

"James, you have *got* to get up!" she said, gently shaking me.

I opened my eyes. Trey was still in the RV, looking sheepish. A second bag of saline had been hooked up while I napped. It was half empty.

"Let me finish my IV," I protested groggily.

"You can finish it on the bike," Sunny said. "In case you've forgotten, we're supposed to be in Alabama tomorrow."

Lucy, who had followed her mother and sister into the RV, chimed in. "*You're* the one who wanted to do this, Dad," she admonished. Trey, a husband, and father also, gave me a knowing look.

By two o'clock I was on my bike, going nowhere inside a twenty-by-fifty-foot workout room with several other bikes set up on either side of me. Darryl occupied the one to my immediate right, Karen the one to his right. Trey also pedaled away on the left.

A steady trickle of supporters came through like attendees of a public viewing to gawk, talk, and take selfies. Each time a phone was raised in front of me, I put on a smile and brandished a fist like a prizefighter. As soon as the shutter clicked, I dropped the fist and the grin. Smiling takes energy.

Around three o'clock, an Asian woman dressed in hospital scrubs walked into the room and came straight up to me. "I just swung by to see how you're doing," she said. "I have to get back to work, so I can't stay. But let me give you my number. Call me if you need anything."

Either this woman knew me, or she thought she knew me, or she was some kind of batty super fan. But I had absolutely no clue who she was.

❸ SHAKE IT OFF

"Um, what do you do?" I asked. "Who are you?"

Her mouth fell open. I saw genuine fear in her eyes, and it made *me* afraid. I still had no clue who she was, but I knew it probably wasn't good that I didn't.

"I'm Jen," the woman said, her voice unsteady. "I'm a doctor. I looked at your hip this morning? I'm probably the only Asian woman in Jackson!"

Nothing.

"I don't remember," I said. "I'm sorry."

Jen left the room looking shattered. I was more than a little shaken myself, but before long I went back to worrying about my aching hip. If it hurt this much on the bike, it would probably be unbearable when I ran. How would I ever get through tonight's marathon?

Then I remembered something. When I was training for the Fifty at home in Utah, my coach, David, would have me use an elliptical trainer—which simulates the running motion but without impact—on days when I was too sore to run. Why not do that now instead of sticking to my plan of running on a treadmill, which merely softens impact without eliminating it? I could gut my way through the Iron Cowboy 5K outside with the local supporters who were already beginning to gather for it, and then come back inside to cover the remaining twenty-three-plus miles without subjecting my wounded body to additional pounding. I called David to ask him what he thought of the plan.

"I think it's a fantastic idea," he said, sounding far more enthusiastic than I'd expected.

Only later would I learn just how relieved David was by my proposal. Since the start of the campaign, he had been sick with worry. At night David tossed and turned, his mind straining to find solutions to my various crises. During the day he consulted with and bounced ideas off specialists of all kinds. Then my bike crash happened, and David really freaked out, convincing himself I would die—literally die—in one horrible way or another if things continued in the direction they were going. Worst of all for him was his powerlessness to do anything to prevent it, so when I called him with my plan to use the elliptical trainer, he pounced on the opportunity to offer counsel that might protect me.

I finished up the ride indoors and then went to the men's locker room to shower and change. When I came out, I bumped into Karen, who had obviously followed me, and who reminded me of my promise to visit the emergency room after my ride. I looked at the time and it was almost eight.

"I can't!" I pleaded. "If I go now, I might as well quit."

Karen looked straight into my eyes for an uncomfortably long time before she spoke again. "I am *telling* you to quit," she said. "You're destroying yourself, James. And for what? It isn't worth it. Please!"

"Oh, it's not that bad," I said, trying to sound breezy. "I think the hardest part is behind me."

I went outside for the 5K wearing a modified left shoe with the toe cut out. (I'd taken some of Karen's advice, at least.) About four dozen people awaited me, including several Ainsley's Angels—runners who push children with disabilities through races in wheelchairs. I'd been so unwaveringly focused on immediate survival during the Fifty that I seldom had any idea who might show up in the next state, but I was happy to see these special participants. I said hello to each of the kids, and then it was time for my daily speech.

The moment I opened my mouth, a lightning storm bore down on us from the west. First came the wind, gusting with enough strength to knock a toddler over. Then the skies burst open, hurling sheets of cold water down on us. The thunderclaps sounded like an aerial bombing, and the lightning flashes appeared in twos and threes. Everyone ran for the door. I hardly needed to say that the Iron Cowboy 5K was canceled.

Inside, I apologized to the group and invited anyone who still wanted to run to follow me to the cardio room, where I chose an elliptical machine and climbed on.

"What are you doing?" Sunny asked.

"I'm going to run on an elliptical today," I said.

"I don't think that's a good idea," she said.

Sunny was considering what I was too survival-focused to consider: elliptical running is *not* a part of the sport of triathlon, and I had told the public I would complete fifty iron-distance *triathlons* in fifty days—not fifty swim-bike-whatevers.

I shrugged my shoulders and began to move, adjusting my pace until my heart rate plateaued at 116 beats per minute, equal to my running heart rate at my usual marathon pace of eleven minutes per mile. After forty-five minutes, my feet went numb. When I stepped off the machine for a potty break, I staggered to the men's room as though I'd been spinning in circles with my eyes closed for the past three-quarters of an hour.

At ten o'clock the club shut down, and we were kicked out. I still had fifteen miles to cover, so we moved the operation to a twenty-four hour fitness club that was located ten miles away. Sariah and her sister Hannah, from ZYTO, laid sleeping bags on the floor of the cardio room and slept. Trey, Darryl, and a couple of others stayed with me, some running on treadmills, others observing, until the very end. We spoke little, but at one point Trey looked at me and shook his head, chuckling.

"Man, what you're doing is amazing," he drawled.

It was approaching two o'clock in the morning when I stepped down from the machine for the last time, feet tingling. The customary finish photo was taken and posted online, along with other photos taken earlier in the evening, that showed me using the elliptical trainer. It never crossed my mind to suppress those images or to worry about how my followers would react to them.

At 6:42 in the morning on Day 20, I was standing on the weather-beaten wooden planks of Fairhope Municipal Pier, gazing out on Mobile Bay. Blustery winds from the west had agitated the cobalt-blue water into a violent froth.

"I'm not swimming in there," I said.

"Good decision," said Johnny, my Alabama ambassador, who owned a triathlon store in town. "Let's find you a pool."

The pool Johnny found for me was located inside a posh private community called the Colony at the Grand. We had to pay to get in, so only Sunny, Casey, and Aaron accompanied me onto the property. I swam by myself with no fanfare, aside from one woman who was a club member. My legs were still tender from the previous day's cramping episode, my right shoulder still killing me.

Aware of my many sore spots, Johnny informed me, as though presenting a gift, that he had mapped out a gentle, mostly flat bike route for me.

"How about *completely* flat?" I asked.

We settled on a ten-mile stretch of Route 98 on the eastern shore of Mobile Bay. The plan was to ride out and back, repeatedly, from a staging area positioned at one end of the route until I'd covered 112 miles. More than twenty local athletes started with me. The course was probably a little boring for them, but it was just what I needed: level, straight, and windless. I settled my forearms into the time-trial bars and watched my spokes spin. Within minutes, I felt my eyelids drooping.

A primal reflex snapped my head up, popped my eyelids open, and sent my heart scudding. I swerved and threw my weight to the left just in time to avoid tipping over. Catastrophe averted, I sat up and checked out my surroundings. I was riding near a large body of water with a bunch of other people, none of whom I recognized.

"Where are we?" I asked the woman closest to me.

"What do you mean?" she answered warily.

"Where is this?" I asked.

"It's called the Eastern Shore Trail," she said.

"I mean which state?"

The woman informed me I was in Fairhope, Alabama, about sixty miles into my Day 20 bike ride. She then drifted back to Johnny, who was riding at the back of our group, and told him what had happened. He instructed his wife, Lisa, and her friend, Katie, to ride on either side of me and talk nonstop for the next fifty miles, and they did.

A stupid math error left me a mile and a half short of 112 when we completed what was supposed to be our last out-and-back. My companions had all had enough and stopped. Johnny needed to organize the Iron Cowboy 5K, so he left too, but not before telling me where to go to knock out the last 1.5 miles. He must have thought I was alert enough now to ride alone, but in fact, my brain was still scrambled. The directions he gave me might as well have been spoken in Mandarin, because my tired brain retained none of it. I set out alone and was lost within minutes. Eventually, I came to a long downslope and coasted to the bottom, where I hit the magic number. On my right stood a church. I swung into the parking lot, dismounted, and called the wingmen for a pickup.

As I was resting inside the motorhome before the start of the run, I used my phone to catch up on social media. On my Facebook page, underneath one of the photos taken during the previous night's marathon, I found a recent comment addressed directly to me.

"Iron Cowboy, did you use an Elliptical trainer to replace a treadmill during the last day or so? If so then you can't, for any reason, say that you have done 19 Ironmans in 19 days and your 50/50/50 is done."

Immediately, I thought of David, who had approved my use of the elliptical machine and who had probably seen this comment, hours earlier. I hurriedly opened up the *Coach's Corner* blog on my Iron Cowboy website. David is a by-the-book kind of guy who is also exceptionally tolerant of criticism, and I felt a dreadful certainty about his reaction to this attack. Sure enough, his recently posted Mississippi write-up delivered a full-throated apology for our decision to use the elliptical. David conceded that my campaign was indeed over in the most official sense. Our stated mission had failed, but he hoped there was still some value in my continuing.

The few comments that had accumulated so far were mostly supportive, but one was gloatingly vicious. Its author, who also addressed me directly, called me a liar and told me to stop embarrassing myself and quit.

Anger gripped me like a sudden fever. I texted David, demanding that he revise and soften his post. But as angry as I was with my coach for halfway siding with my critics, I was far more furious with myself for having handed them a gift-wrapped opportunity to pile on the criticism. How could I not have seen this coming? Sunny clearly had, and she'd tried to warn me. Why hadn't I listened?

I burned with frustration at my inability to go back in time and heed my wife's counsel. There was no doubt in my mind that I could have run, or at least walked yesterday's marathon. It was hardly an excuse to avoid tough circumstances, being that I had run the marathon the night of the crash, in much worse condition. I hadn't used the elliptical machine out of necessity, I'd used it because it seemed to me that running on an elliptical machine at 116 beats per minute was more in the spirit of my quest, at that moment, than was the alternative of walking on a treadmill or outdoors at 96 BPM. It certainly wasn't easier; it was just safer. My numb feet reminded me that logging 26.2 miles, or 6 hours, on an elliptical, is not easier or more enjoyable than running that same distance. I found it to be far more mentally challenging and just as physically uncomfortable.

I stepped out of the motorhome to start my run in a black mood. I thought of the 26.2 miles in front of me, and of the thirty more triathlons yet to come. What was the point? Even if I survived them, there was already an asterisk next to my achievement that could never be erased. I felt as if a trapdoor had opened under me. The one thing I needed most in order to see this thing through was hunger, an absolute conviction that achieving my goal would be worth all the suffering. In an instant, that flame of desire had been snuffed.

We were staging in a part of Fairhope called the Windmill Market, a kind of upscale bazaar featuring farm-to-fork restaurants, a local foods grocer, and craft shops, all powered by solar panels and a windmill. When I returned there after taking an initial three-mile bite out of my marathon, I discovered a large and energized crowd waiting to join me for the 5K. Their enthusiastic presence should have given me a boost, but instead, it only deepened my despondency. For the next hour, I had to be "on," smiley and chatty when all I really wanted to do was crawl into a hole.

I continued to brood on what David, in his blog post, had glibly dubbed El-liptigate, as I ran into the night with the eight or ten locals who elected to hang on with me after the 5K. What bothered me most was my critics' insinuation that I was trying to evade the challenge I had created for myself. This charge was so thoroughly unjustified, and it so badly misrepresented who I was and what I stood for that I wanted to punch a hole in a wall. My intention in planning and starting the Fifty had never been to set an official world record; it was to discover the limits of my physical and mental endurance and to *Redefine Impossible.* In the end, I didn't care what anyone else thought. All I cared about was reaching my breaking point and seeing what happened when I got there. The trolls and haters seemed to believe that if I completed the campaign having taken the easy way out, but I was the only one who knew it, I would be satisfied. They couldn't have been more wrong.

Then again, I *did* care what other people thought—not the people who wanted me to fail, but those who wanted me to succeed. After all, if the only thing that con-cerned me was finding my limit, I could have done it without the hoopla of the Fifty. I'd chosen to draw attention to my quest because I wanted to affect people. Over the past twenty days, I had been pleasantly surprised, not so much by how many people I was reaching, but by the kinds of people the campaign was drawing into its orbit. The Guinness World Records I'd set in 2010 and 2012 for the most half-iron-dis-tance triathlons completed in one year (twenty-two) and the most full iron-distance triathlons completed in one year (thirty) had mostly impressed other athletes, but my current undertaking was going way beyond that.

Just that morning, before my bike ride, I received a fist bump from a little boy of about my son Quinn's age. His father, Doug, a recently recovered drug addict, and a single parent had decided to show his son a vision for a better life by taking him on an epic Iron Cowboy–themed road trip. I would see them in seven states, and after-ward, Doug would tell me, "The ripple effect of your commitment and choice to do what you have done is infinite."

I thought about the people I had met in earlier states who had surmounted can-cer, obesity, paralysis, and other huge obstacles and were excited about my mission as a kind of universal symbol of overcoming adversity. Something about my attempt to *Redefine Impossible* seemed to empower people to achieve their own personal *im-possible.*

Then I thought of Trey from Mississippi. A latecomer to the sport of triathlon, Trey had found in it more joy and fulfillment than he had found previously in any occupation, hobby, or pastime. It had awakened the dreamer in him. From talking to Trey last night, I'd learned that he saw me as a fellow dreamer who wasn't afraid to go for it, and my example inspired him to do the same. Trey had said to me, "Man, what you're doing is amazing," *while I was on the elliptical trainer.* Clearly, it made no difference to him that I'd chosen a nonimpact machine instead of a treadmill. Nor did it seem to have made any difference to the dozens of Alabamans who had ridden their bikes and run with me today, none of whom had even mentioned the scandal hanging over me.

Screw the haters, I decided. This campaign was *not* over. Heck, I was still pushing my body and mind further than I ever had, and perhaps as far as any athlete ever had. I was still doing the impossible and empowering others to do their impossible. How foolish would it be for me to allow my critics to rob me of the motivation I needed to finish what I had started? Instead of giving them what they wanted, I would use the anger they had stoked in me to redouble my hunger to succeed. From that moment forward, I vowed to myself that I would give the trolls and haters no more ammunition with which to discredit me. Not one bit.

I ran every step of the marathon in Alabama. Despite the continuing pain in my hip and toe, I refused to walk, taking grim pleasure in my newly adopted I'll-show-you frame of mind.

We were cruising along Fairhope Avenue with less than a mile to go when a sudden commotion in the darkness startled us. Two nearly naked men leaped out from the bushes, whooping and hollering and waving their arms. It was the wingmen, wearing Iron Cowboy speedos, running shoes, and nothing else. Music blared from Casey's phone—Taylor Swift's "Shake It Off."

And the haters gonna hate, hate, hate, hate, hate
Baby, I'm just gonna shake, shake, shake, shake, shake
I shake it off. I shake it off

The wingmen pranced and whirled ahead of us as the maddeningly infectious pop song played on, and my supporters laughed themselves dizzy. The effect on me was a bit more delayed. Unmoved initially, I was laughing right along with everyone else when the performance ended. The wingmen and I had not discussed the latest scuttlebutt, nor would we, but I knew they knew about it, and they must have known how it was affecting me. There was great love and—I had to admit—a certain brilliance in the scheme they had concocted to take my mind off the negativity pressing down on me from cyberspace.

Haters gonna hate, James. Shake it off.

Day 20 came to an end outside Johnny's store. I took a quick shower in the back of the shop while Aaron rummaged for food inside the motor home, which was now parked outside, bringing a freshly awakened Sunny back with him. Clean and dry, I lay down on a massage table to receive an adjustment from Ryan, a local chiropractor. Sunny and Katie (the same Katie who had helped keep me awake during my last fifty miles on the bike) massaged my legs as Ryan dug deep into my neck.

I followed the others' conversation for a short while with my eyes closed and then fell asleep. I only know what happened next because my video crew was also present. The clip they filmed shows me snoring peacefully with my head resting in the hands of an incredulous Ryan, who had never seen a person fall asleep during an adjustment and would have sworn it wasn't possible. To see if I was faking, Ryan let my head drop lifelessly off the edge of the table, but the snoring continued. This invited a few snickers, but when I first watched the clip, I thought I detected a note of uneasiness in the laughter of those who'd only met me that day.

One thing is certain: none of them thought they were looking at a man who wanted the easy way out.

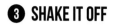

❸ SHAKE IT OFF

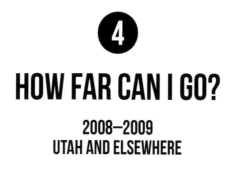

HOW FAR CAN I GO?

2008–2009
UTAH AND ELSEWHERE

One of the worst jobs you could have when the Great Recession hit in 2008 was the one I had: a mortgage lender. Count me among the tens of thousands of saps who got sucked up in the hysteria of the real estate bubble and changed careers in the hope of emulating the success of those fortunate enough to have already been in the housing industry when the bonanza began.

In my case, there was a family influence at play as well. Sunny's dad was a commercial real estate developer, one of her brothers was a general contractor, and two of her sisters worked as real estate agents. In 2006, they began to tell me—half-jokingly at first—that I ought to become a mortgage lender, in order to complete the vertical integration of the Hatfield (Sunny's maiden name) real estate empire. Having no room for advancement at Copeland's Sports, I took a course, got licensed, and processed my first loan in February 2007.

It started out well. I had a vast local network, people skills, and market winds at my back. Before long, I was bringing in more business than I could handle, so my friend Rob and I opened our own business, Elevate Home Loans on State Street in Orem. By March 2008, I had five loan officers and three processors working under me.

Then the Bear Stearns investment firm collapsed. I had a client's loan application in underwriting at the time, and it fell through—unheard of during the brief time I'd been in business. Almost overnight, the banks had gone from reckless to skittish. *The beginning of the end,* I thought, and it was. Three months later, I shut the doors on Elevate Home Loans.

The timing couldn't have been worse. Our fourth daughter, Dolly, had just been born in January, and Sunny was pregnant again. We were living in a six-bedroom house on the Seven Peaks Resort Golf Course in Provo, and having our dream home built in nearby Lindon—a 5,500-square-foot, seven-bedroom mini-mansion with a wraparound porch. Our monthly nut for the two mortgages came to $7,500.

I had a high school education and no particular skills beyond a low-single-digit golf handicap. We all knew that the real estate market wasn't going to turn around and I needed income badly. I picked up several sales jobs, but when those companies shut down, I never received my commission paychecks. I needed any work I could get, so I worked in a call center, built kitchen cabinets, and did construction cleanup. But the work was spotty, and it never came close to covering our fixed costs.

As the months ticked by and our savings dwindled, Sunny and I took increasingly desperate measures. We started with low-hanging fruit, like canceling our cable television service. Sunny, despite having four children below the age of five to look after, and a fifth on the way, started babysitting and doing any other odd jobs she could do for pay. I sold off all the toys I had acquired while working at Copeland's: golf clubs, skis, snowboards, kayaks, backpacks, etc. I put so much stuff up for sale on eBay that company watchdogs flagged me as a possible thief!

We racked up credit card debt just to survive. This was in hopes that when our other house sold, we could pay the debt off and get our finances back in order. We made partial payments on various bills, and then we finally applied for food stamps. That last one hurt as much as it helped. My face burned with shame the first time I selected the EBT payment option on a supermarket checkout console. I had been an American citizen for just one year (I was slow to apply), and I had already become a parasite (as I saw myself) to the country that had opened its arms to me.

Our great hope for financial salvation was selling our house in Provo, but we might as well have been trying to sell a rocket ship in Amish Country. When our dream home was completed in 2009, we moved into it anyway, leaving it mostly unfurnished. By this time, I knew bankruptcy was our only way out. Sunny, however, refused to accept it.

"I don't want to quit until we really have no other options," she said.

"You tell me when you're ready," I told her.

One evening I was at home, the day was done and our family was relaxing before the kids went to bed. Lucy came to me and said, "Dad, a creepy man is snooping around outside." I fetched my 9mm semiautomatic pistol and stuffed it in the waistband of my pants at the small of my back, then flung open the front door. Sure enough, a thuggish-looking dude with a burly bouncer's body was trying to peer into our garage.

"Get off my property," I said by way of greeting.

The man turned toward me calmly and smiled like a movie villain.

"Why don't you pay your bills, man?" he asked.

Repo man, of course.

He tried to humiliate us, threatening to talk to our neighbors and expose us. But our neighbors were close friends and family, and even if they weren't, we wouldn't care. This guy was just trying to be a jerk. Lucy's fear had brought out the Tarzan in me. If I was part Tarzan, my antagonist was a gorilla through and through, and he clearly enjoyed our escalating verbal battle, and this pissed me off even more. I would have regretted shooting him, but not right away.

When the repo man left, I went back inside and told Sunny what had happened. Three days later, we removed the child safety seats from our Toyota Highlander and returned it to the dealership.

Sunny and I often huddled together in our fabulous dream kitchen crunching numbers. The ritual followed the same script each time, ending with me voting for bankruptcy and Sunny advocating for patience. But our next session was different, "We can't go on like this," Sunny said, "I'm ready."

I felt relief as immense as that of a plummeting skydiver whose backup parachute opens just in time. I also felt freedom: the freedom of realizing I had nothing left to lose. Then there was hope, a refreshing chance at a fresh start.

I had hated being a mortgage lender. It combined all the things I most despised: numbers, paperwork, offices, and sitting still. Worse, I spent way too much time doing it—sixty hours a week away from Sunny and the kids. On top of that, it was an utterly thankless job. I could put together the juiciest deal ever for a client, and he would still assume I was ripping him off somehow. I had no control because success depended not on skill or hard work, but the health of the economy.

I died a little each time I walked into my office on State Street. The only thing that could have been worse for me than losing the business was keeping it, continuing to process loans year after soul-sucking year, until I put myself out to pasture. I was not challenging myself, exercising my gifts, or making any meaningful contribution to the world.

Life wasn't all bad, though. I was thankful for so many things in my life. My wife and children, who brought me great joy and a deep sense of purpose. I also had mounds of friends, and I loved living in Utah; but I knew that something was missing; family, friends, and a pleasant environment just weren't enough. To be truly happy, I also needed a calling—a career or mission that fit my nature, took me on an adventure, and allowed me to make my mark in the world. I didn't want to die knowing I had lived only half of a life. I was now well into my thirties, almost half-way through life, and I felt that the dreamer in me was on life support. The decision to file for bankruptcy afforded me one last chance to find my true calling. But what was it?

Rewind with me for a minute to 2005. In the summer after the wheelchair in-cident at the E Center that left me with a searing need to prove my toughness, I completed fourteen short-course triathlons. I chose to do multisport races instead of more marathons because I enjoyed the variety of training and competing in three disciplines. I soon discovered after I bought a cheap cyclo-cross bike, to use in my first triathlon, that I especially loved cycling. My long training rides in Provo Can-yon became my Zen time, an escape from the noise of reality into a flow state where I became one with my body's exertions and the surrounding environment.

Endurance sports are a slippery slope. The more time you invest in them, the more you improve, and the more improvement, the more motivated you are to keep pushing. Triathlons certainly don't appeal to everyone, but they scratch an itch for those who find a kind of spiritual satisfaction in pushing their physical and mental limits. Progress in this journey is like a drug; it feels good, but it's never enough. I got hooked quickly, racing every single weekend in the summer of 2005 with no intention of slowing down.

And I did improve. By 2006 I was well-known on the Utah triathlon scene, a man to beat in local races, never failing to make the podium in my age group, often winning my category, and occasionally winning races outright. In 2007, I completed my first half-iron-distance triathlon and the following year my first full Ironman.

I sensed it was all leading somewhere, but I didn't know exactly where. I was a little too old and a bit too slow to turn professional. My best Olympic-distance tri-athlon time of 1:56 would have made me a world champion if I had been a woman,

❹ HOW FAR CAN I GO?

but the top men were ten minutes faster. If I wanted to distinguish myself, I would have to blaze my own trail.

Experience had taught me that what I lacked in speed, I made up for in durability. I wasn't unbreakable, but when I did break down, I bounced back quickly. My greatest strength, however, was my mind. In the early days, I took for granted the quitting-is-not-an-option mentality I brought to the racecourse, but over time I came to see that most endurance athletes, even most successful ones, weren't the type of people who could ride a Ferris wheel continuously for ten days. This combination of physical durability and mental resilience suggested a unique kind of potential. Perhaps my quest was not to see how fast I could go, but how far.

In 2009, around the time my last child, Quinn, was born, Sunny's father, Ron, offered me a job with his charity, In Our Own Quiet Way, which funded water retention systems in Kenya. The gesture was his way of helping me without hurting my pride. I worked in the corporate division, trying to drum up commercial sponsorships. Ron said he was open to new ideas, and I took him at his word. Inspiration struck during one of my rides in Provo Canyon. Aware that people often used feats of endurance to raise money for charities, I thought, *Why don't I do that?* I wondered what the record was for the most official Ironman triathlons completed in one year.

A phone call to Guinness revealed the answer: twenty. That was formidable. I had completed only one Ironman ever, but during the same call, I learned there was no record for half-iron-distance triathlons. It made sense—a kind of sense, anyway—to start there and, if all went well, move up.

I ran the idea by Sunny during "quiet time"—the period between eight o'clock p.m. and bedtime when the kids had to leave Mommy and Daddy alone so they could talk about adult stuff. As half-baked and impractical as my scheme might have seemed, Sunny supported it without hesitation.

"I believe in you," she said. "Besides, what else are you going to do—go back to school and pile up a bunch of student debt so you can get some other job you hate?"

The next day we made the pitch to Ron in our kitchen, and he rubber-stamped it. We named the project Tri and Give a Dam. My charge was to raise enough money to build twenty dams in Kenya by breaking the nonexistent Guinness World Record for the most half-iron-distance triathlons completed in one year.

I did not doubt my ability to complete twenty such races (Guinness's minimum requirement for record certification) in the 2010 calendar year. The hard part would be financing the venture. I began calling and visiting local businesses, asking each

45

of them to pony up the entry fee (about $300) for one race. A surprising number of them went for it. I canvassed companies in the endurance space and begged for free stuff, meeting with similar success. Ellsworth gave me a bike, Blue Seventy a wetsuit, Altra a steady supply of running shoes, and Young Living all the essential oils I wanted, in addition to paying to build a dam in Africa. I hit up friends and associates for donations of unused airline miles and hotel rewards points. In a word, I got resourceful.

The record attempt began in Oceanside, California, on March 27, 2010. Race number one went off without a hitch. Our friends Garen and Debbie decided to join us on this first trip, making it a couple's vacation. I completed the race in a respectable time of 5 hours and 5 minutes. Barring unforeseen crises, this thing was going to be a cakewalk.

My first unforeseen crisis occurred in June, on my return home from Ironman 70.3 Hawaii, my sixth race. In that event, I had ridden a one-of-a-kind prototype of a new Ellsworth triathlon bike. The company had loaned the machine to me with the caution that it was irreplaceable *and* must be returned in the same mint condition in which I had received it. I was standing at the oversized baggage collection point at Salt Lake City International Airport, waiting for my bike case to appear, when I heard my name over the PA system. The voice instructed me to go to the Delta baggage claim counter, where I was met by a plump woman in her mid-forties.

"I'm afraid there was a small incident involving your checked item, Mr. Lawrence," she said. "We just need you to take a look at it and make sure everything is okay." I felt my bowels loosen. The woman led me into a back room that looked like a graveyard for lost luggage. I didn't see my bike case anywhere among the beat-up-looking bags, boxes, and crates strewn about. When my escort gestured toward it, I realized why. It was totally unrecognizable, just a pile of black plastic debris. I sifted through the wreckage and discovered that the bike itself, was in the same state, smashed to smithereens.

"You're going to pay for this, right?" I asked.

"I'm afraid not," the woman said primly. "You signed a waiver releasing the airline from liability."

"I paid $200 to check it," I said. "You're at least going to give me a refund."

"Actually, no," the woman said. "We don't do refunds."

Unbelievable! I needed that money! I was supposed to race again the very next weekend in Boise, and now I had no bike to use. But this worry paled in comparison to my dread of informing the generous people at Ellsworth that their prototype had been run over and destroyed on my watch. I left the airport feeling angrier than I had since—since when?—since I'd caught the repo man peeking into my garage! The next morning I sat down in front of my computer and filmed a video rant.

"Hey, there," I began. "My name's James Lawrence. I'm an athlete with the Tri and Give a Dam project, and I just got screwed by Delta Airlines." Stretching my production skills, I included a photo montage of the destroyed bike and bike case, setting it to the Lionel Richie / Diana Ross duet "Endless Love."

"What am I going to do now, Delta?" I concluded. "How am I going to race this weekend? What about the kids in Africa?"

I uploaded the video to YouTube and promptly forgot about it, turning my attention to the pressing matter of finding a new bike for Boise. While I slept that night, the video went viral, amassing 80,000 views in twenty-four hours, and the following afternoon I received a call from a PR executive at Delta. She asked me if I would kindly take down the video while a solution was negotiated. In the end, the company agreed to refund my checked-luggage fee and compensate Ellsworth for the loss of their prototype. Now was that so hard?

On Saturday, I competed in my seventh race of the year on a bike I borrowed from my friend Jess. Fired up by my recent victory over corporate tyranny, I not only finished the race, but also managed to qualify for the Ironman 70.3 World Championship, which was to be held in Clearwater, Florida at the end of the year.

Throughout the spring and into the summer I looked forward to August 28, when I was scheduled to participate in the Utah Half, in Provo, with Sunny. It would be her first half-iron-distance triathlon and the first triathlon of any kind that we did together. We slept in our own bed the night before the race, a nice departure from the stale-smelling budget hotel rooms, complete strangers' beds (I had become a master of the "homestay"), and rental cars I'd slept in before previous events. My plan was to swim as fast as I could on behalf of an Aquaphor-sponsored relay team that I had joined, then wait for Sunny in the transition area and complete the bike and run segments of the race with her.

One thing that I had learned, in the process of acquiring a lot of racing experience, in a compressed period of time, was that you never knew what you were going to experience at each race when the starting horn sounded. On the morning of the Utah Half race, I realized that my experience wasn't going to be pleasant. The rough day started when half-way through the swim, a woman who had started five minutes behind me, in the following group, passed me *breast-stroking.*

I reached the transition area and found that the bike racked next to mine, owned by a 220-pound former Brigham Young University running back named Joe, was gone. *Oh, no!* I thought. *Someone stole Joe's bike!* That someone, it turned out, was Joe, who had unexpectedly outswam me and was already well up the road.

Sunny, all smiles, came into the transition area and we rolled out on our bikes with our friend and massage therapist, Natalie. Eight miles in, I flatted, so Sunny suggested she and Natalie ride ahead while I fixed it. I approved the idea, knowing I would have no trouble catching up to her.

It took thirty miles of all-out effort to chase her down. Apparently, Sunny had been training while I was crisscrossing the continent collecting finisher medals. By the time I caught up, I was toast. With five miles left to ride, I felt a scary twinge in my right hamstring. When I dismounted, I immediately knew that I would not be able to run, and I told Sunny to go ahead. I couldn't afford to risk blowing the rest of the season by forcing it today, because this was only race sixteen. I called Jess—the guy who'd loaned me his bike for Boise—to let him know not to look for me out on the run course.

"Who is this?" Jess asked. "I thought I was talking to James Lawrence. There must be some mistake because the James Lawrence I know *doesn't quit!* Man, all you have to do is walk! It'll take forever, but who cares? This is for a world record! And if you quit now and break the record anyway, do you really want a DNF [Did Not Finish] on your résumé? You've already done the swim and the bike. Heck, I'll come down there and walk with you. Just do it!"

Duly chastened, I accepted Jess's challenge, and after three hours and eighteen minutes of surprisingly enjoyable limping (I seemed to know every third person I saw on the road), triathlon number sixteen was in the books.

Two weeks later, I competed in Muskoka, Ontario, and my hamstring was already 90 percent improved. I would go on to complete a total of twenty-two half-iron-distance triathlons before the year was out and become a certified Guinness World Record holder. Inside that record was the only race where Sunny had officially beat me. She would never let me forget that in the one race we did together, she beat me by an hour.

My last event was the Ironman 70.3 World Championship in Clearwater, Florida. Sunny, Ron, and Sunny's mom, Maurine, came out for it. I had another hard day, a nasty new pain in my left iliotibial band reducing me to intermittent walking during the half marathon. After the race, I met up with Sunny and her parents inside a VIP tent located just beyond the finish line. We sat at a plastic table—I still in my sweaty race uniform—and toasted my achievement with free finger foods, lacking the funds to dine at a proper restaurant.

I tried to be fully present and enjoy the moment, but part of my mind was elsewhere, looking ahead. The mission I had just completed had been intended to serve as a steppingstone, and that's exactly what it felt like, I felt unfulfilled. I had hoped to raise enough money to build twenty dams and had fallen nineteen dams short. There had been a few decent media hits—short pieces on Ironman.com and Yahoo News among them—but I had a lot to learn about the science of self-promotion. Above all, the challenge itself had been hard but not *that* hard, and the knowledge and experience I had gained in the process of completing it left me feeling ready—and hungry—for more.

I still had no idea where this strange path I had chosen would ultimately lead, I just knew I hadn't gotten there yet. Not even close.

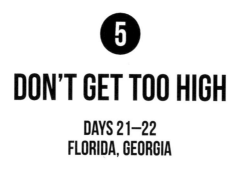

5

DON'T GET TOO HIGH

DAYS 21–22
FLORIDA, GEORGIA

Casey steered the motorhome into the brick driveway of Evan's brick house in north Pensacola at two-thirty in the morning on Day 21. A porch light came on, and my Florida co-ambassador came out.

"What time do we need to leave tomorrow?" Casey asked him.

"You mean today," Evan corrected. "Be ready in two hours."

Casey decided it wasn't worth the bother to wake me up and transfer me to Evan's guest bed, but he knew I would not be happy when I opened my eyes to find myself on the same thin mattress where I'd fallen asleep. Tonight was meant to have been my first, and only chance, in all fifty days to sleep eight hours in a proper bed, as Pensacola was less than sixty miles away from our last stop in Fairhope, Alabama. I had looked forward to this opportunity since the start of the campaign, ever more so as my sufferings piled up. Unfortunately, a late finish on Day 20 followed by a lengthy pit stop (full septic tank) off Route 10, had blown that chance.

Aaron shook me awake at Pensacola Beach at sunrise. Casey was right—I wasn't happy. Sunny took my hand and escorted me to a pavilion, where a massage therapist was waiting. I laid on the table and was instantly asleep. Ninety minutes later, I was reawakened, and Sunny led me by the hand to the beach. "I know you are tired, My Love. I let the massage therapist go 90 minutes so that you could sneak in a little extra sleep." This gesture was unusual for Sunny, as she was the one trying her best to get us back on schedule. I am sure that her senses told her that I needed it today.

I was standing on the powdery sand of Pensacola Beach next to Ricki, a pretty young blond woman, wearing a bright blue dress, and holding a fat microphone. Ricki spoke directly to a tripod-mounted camera for a few seconds and then turned to me.

"How has it been so far?" she asked.

"I'm tired," I said.

My voice was thin and ragged, and my eyes were slits.

"Well," Ricki said, thrown off by my brevity, "you're doing a great job; and it's all for a great cause, right?"

Suddenly I felt an overwhelming urge to cry. My eyes welled up, and there was a long, awkward pause. Then I nodded, giggled lightly, and whispered, "Yeah."

Evan and his friend John, my other co-ambassador, were watching from the wings. Both of them thought I had briefly lost consciousness on live television. The segment was later posted on Facebook. The first comment was this:

He did not seem right in his interview this morning. I hope that he has some-one attending [to] his medical needs and will have the ability to stop him from hurting himself.

The only thing I remember about the rest of the interview is poor Ricki's frozen facial expression. She looked as though she had just eaten something foul-tasting and had to pretend to like it.

As soon as Ricki released me, I strode into the ocean, where Sunny waited, ankle-deep. She rubbed my arm and spoke soothingly. "It's like bathwater," she said. "I think you're going to enjoy this one."

The Santa Rosa Sound's warm brine is stunningly clear and on days like this one, as smooth as a mirror. I swam back and forth along a course marked by buoys, set out just for me in five feet of water, guided by a paddleboarder and two strong swimmers, and followed by a pod of local triathletes. Through the fog of sleepiness, I slowly became aware that aside from my still-aching right shoulder, my body felt powerful and fresh, as though I hadn't swum in a few days. When I paused to check my distance, I was swimming at almost the same pace I do in actual races. Where had this person been the last couple weeks?

On the fifth lap, now fully awake and almost cheerful, I was going to hit 2.4 miles well before I got back to where I'd started, so I veered toward shore. My fingertips were scraping bottom when my watch displayed the desired number. I stood up, all around me were heads bobbing in bemused silence. I felt like Forrest Gump at the moment he quit running.

"I'll walk from here," I said. "I don't swim a yard more than I have to."

Back on the beach, I rinsed the salt off my body in a cold outdoor shower and went inside the motorhome, where John and his friend Scott, a local triathlete who owned a bunch of Subway restaurants, brought breakfast sandwiches for everyone. I enjoyed three or four.

Santa Rosa Island is a thread like strip of land, twenty-eight miles long and barely 400 meters wide. Recent storms had washed out parts of its one major road, so John and Evan hastily changed my bike course to a ten-mile out-and-back, which was fine by me. We relocated the vehicles to a spot that was slightly less overrun by tourists on this hot Saturday in the Florida Panhandle's peak tourist season, and I set out from there with more than twenty supporters. The splendor of my surroundings seeped into my soul as we wheeled back and forth along Route 399. The sparkling ocean was visible over both shoulders, just a stone's throw away in either direction. The beaches became increasingly alive with American summer culture—kites, coolers, sand castles, bikinis, and all the rest.

My only complaint was the air. The heavy winds out of the west turned the ride into a de facto interval workout. When I pedaled east, a friendly invisible shove from the rear did half the work for me. When I turned around, a cruel push from the front tossed sand in my gears, or it seemed that way. My mood fluctuated in a matching rhythm. Riding with the wind, I was content; riding against the wind, I was deflated. This pattern did not, at the time, strike me as an allegory for the campaign as a whole, much less as a warning.

I was riding into the wind on my sixth out-and-back when my friend Kyle came cruising toward me on my spare bike. He had just flown in from Utah for a short stint with the campaign (his second). He swung around and sidled up next to me.

"You look great!" he said, surprised. I had looked far from great when he had last seen me in Colorado.

"I *feel* great," I said. "What a difference a day makes!"

On the last lap—again riding against the wind—I sped up. A kind of bodily euphoria had taken hold of me, a survivor's bliss fueled by a sense of having come out the other side of a spirit-testing ordeal. Underneath the tiredness and soreness, I discovered, I was still incredibly fit...go figure.

My unexpected acceleration put several of my companions, including Kyle, under pressure. By the time I got back to the staging area, only three or four riders were still with me.

IRON COWBOY

I handed over my bike to Casey, tore off my cycling jersey, and led my kids into the ocean, where we sat in the shallows and soaked. It was the first moment of real daddy time I'd had with them since the start of the campaign. Scott, the Subway guy, had taken them out on his powerboat for a few hours while I was riding. I heard all about the nineteenth-century military fort they'd checked out and the dolphins that had swum next to them on the boat. As I squinted into the sun and let their precious voices wash over me, I could almost imagine we were a normal family like any other, that we had nothing more to do today than grill some burgers and dogs and sit around on beach chairs, talking and laughing. It pained me almost physically to tear myself away from the five of them and get ready to run.

The afternoon had turned into a scorcher. When I started running with Evan and a dozen others at four thirty, it was eighty-nine degrees and tropically humid. Moving eastward with the wind felt like running under a giant magnifying glass.

"This isn't going to work," I said to Evan after the first mile.

He gave me a panicked look. Evan and John had taken total responsibility for providing the conditions I needed to complete today's triathlon successfully. I had more or less just asked Evan to change the weather.

Moments later, we passed a house with an open garage and a man tinkering away at something inside. A member of our group peeled off and approached him, asking questions I wasn't able to overhear. He rejoined us brandishing a black-and-white-striped umbrella, which he opened and held over me as we ran. The relief was immediate. My supporters took turns shading me until we turned around and the abrupt switch from a headwind to tailwind transformed the umbrella into an uncontrollable flyaway risk and stabbing hazard. The instrument was returned to its owner the next time we passed his house.

The staging area had become a mob scene during our ninety-minute absence. Supporters were lined up at our merchandise table, children scampered around like puppies at a dog park, and local endurance community members stood in circles, chatting. I picked my way through the crowd and bumped into Dallas, who had just come in from the airport. My old friend and trusted body mechanic eyed my gait and frowned.

"You're limping," he observed.

"Well, that's a relief," I said.

"A relief? What do you mean?"

"I thought I was just imagining it."

54

❺ DON'T GET TOO HIGH

Dallas gestured toward the portable treatment table we traveled with, and I laid down. His familiar touch soothed my mind even before it repaired my body. With sure movements of his experienced hands, Dallas tested the affected tissues, discovering in no time that the muscles surrounding my damaged right hip had effectively shut down in a protective response to pain, putting a hitch in my giddy-up. I could feel those muscles reawakening as he worked them over.

Evan came by and tapped his wrist with two fingers to signal it was time to get the Iron Cowboy 5K under way. He led me to a folding table with a speaker on top and placed a microphone in my hand. Passing beachgoers hearing my amplified voice, and seeing the crowd gathered around me, stopped to listen. One or two of them even bought Iron Cowboy T-shirts, despite still having only the vaguest notion of who I was.

We attracted more attention on the move, our happy clan trotting westward toward a pinkening horizon along streets choked with creeping vehicles, music blaring from some, others acknowledging us with a friendly tap of the horn. The sidewalks teemed with pedestrians on their way to restaurants and nightclubs, barbecues and bonfires. I heard a few shouts of, "Go, Iron Cowboy!"—perhaps from people who'd seen my bizarre interview with Ricki that morning.

A young serviceman named Billy had come all the way from Biloxi to run with me. At the start of my marathon, Billy had told me he was going to run the whole thing. After the 5K, our group now down to fewer than a dozen, he spoke to me again.

"I heard you like hamburgers," he said.

"You heard right," I said.

"You want one now?" he asked.

"I think I do."

Billy called in an order to Tops Choice Hamburgers. I requested a plain burger with lettuce and pickles and sweet potato fries on the side. Billy even convinced the person who took the order to send a server out to the roadside to wait for us. When we came up to her, Billy snatched the bag from her hand, and we ate our burgers and fries on the go. In retrospect, I wish I'd asked Billy if he had ever run while eating a burger. Soon after he swallowed his last bite, he staggered to a halt, hands on his stomach. That's the last I saw of him.

At ten o'clock, I made one last stop at the staging area to say goodbye to Sunny and the kids before they took off for Atlanta. I got another quick treatment from

Dallas, scarfed some food, and then, conscious of time, rejoined my surviving supporters to complete Day 21.

"Okay, we've got eight miles to go," Evan said.

"Seven point nine miles," I corrected.

"I thought we stopped at 18.2," he said.

"We did. But I've walked a tenth of a mile since then," I said. "I never stopped my watch."

Evan looked at me as though he were about to give me grief but then thought better of it, perhaps realizing he'd probably do the same in my shoes.

Everyone took turns sharing their stories as we logged those last 7.9 miles. One woman had dragged her husband all the way from Louisiana on their wedding anniversary so she could run with me. Another had recently lost 150 pounds. Her voice thickened as she told us how important it was to her to set a positive example for her children. After she had told her husband about my journey, he was ecstatic and was finally showing interest in changing his lifestyle.

My reward for completing triathlon number twenty-one was another cold outdoor shower. Evan hustled me along, fearful of ruining the day's success at the last moment by failing to deliver me to the next venue on schedule.

Only Dallas and Kyle had stayed behind to accompany me on the long drive to Atlanta. The three of us took our places inside the van—Kyle behind the wheel, I on my sleeping pallet, and Dallas beside me, ready to begin a sequence of treatments that would take almost two hours to complete. By the time he switched off the cold laser (a device used to treat pain and promote tissue healing), the van smelled like a locker room and my bedding was soaked from melted ice. I smelled nothing, felt nothing.

Each morning there came a terrible moment when, having achieved a certain level of wakefulness, I remembered with sickening dread what lay before me. On Day 22, that moment occurred at six thirty, as Dallas and Kyle spoke my name and shook my shoulders trying to wake me up for my swim at Life Time Fitness in Mountain Brook, Georgia. A childish rage boiled up inside me.

"Just leave me alone!" I barked.

Dallas and Kyle laughed, and my anger increased.

⑤ DON'T GET TOO HIGH

"Touch me again, and I swear I'll punch you in the face!" I bellowed.

Dallas and Kyle howled in delight.

Sunny and the wingmen arrived at the swim location and caught a short nap. Jason, my Georgia ambassador, was there and ready to be my support/friend for the day. Sunny climbed inside the van, spoke softly, and stroked my cheeks. Seeing an opportunity, Casey and Aaron crowded inside with us and wagged their butts in my face and blew in my ears.

"There's a woman here to give you a massage," Sunny said. "Why don't you come outside so Renee can work on you before you swim?"

"Tell her to come in here," I said.

Sunny seized on the compromise and in a moment Renee took the place of Sunny and the wingmen. After three weeks on the road, I considered myself a connoisseur of bodywork. I knew what I liked and what I didn't like, and few massage therapists met my high standards. I wasn't expecting much from this Renee person, but I felt the magic in her fingers from the very first touch.

"Let's move to the table," I told her.

I crawled out of the van and lay face down on the treatment table to allow Renee to do her job properly. Within seconds I was snoring.

Eventually, I had no choice but to get up and get ready to swim. Flanking me like prison guards, Sunny and the crew marched me inside the Life Time Fitness building and right up to the edge of the pool, as though I might make a run for it. I looked over and saw Matt and Bonnie, Sunny's cousins. They happened to be traveling in the area and came to offer support. It was comforting to see familiar faces, especially for Sunny. She had worked through this journey with little or no support, and now there was family; her smile was as wide as her face. I turned back to the water's edge, feeling like a pirate's captive being made to walk the plank. I did not so much jump in as fall into the water.

While I swam, a cloudburst dumped a good old Southern rain outside. Kyle and the wingmen huddled with Jason (who had cycled with me in Chattanooga and had witnessed my crash, which he did not care to see repeated on his watch) and made the decision for me to ride indoors. When I heard these plans, I gave them an emphatic thumbs-down. I didn't care if the forecasters were calling for a 100 percent chance of simultaneous hurricanes, tornadoes, earthquakes, and wildfires, I would ride outside no matter what. I was determined not to give the Internet trolls and haters more rope with which to hang me.

IRON COWBOY

Jason's friend Elizabeth, who had also ridden with me in Chattanooga, brought breakfast for everyone: bacon, pancakes, *bacon pancakes,* breakfast burritos, and eggs. While we ate, Jason laid out plan B, which entailed a twenty-five-mile relocation to the Silver Comet Trail, an extensive rail trail stretching westward from Smyrna to the Alabama state line. Renee gave me a second award-worthy massage during the drive over to our new staging area. We arrived there to find more than fifty people waiting, about half of them with bikes.

My first look at the Silver Comet Trail sent my spirits soaring. In front of me laid an asphalt path as smooth and flat like a frog pond, snaking gently between tall trees providing total shade. Typically jammed with cyclists, walkers, and joggers on a Sunday in June, it was virtually empty today—aside from the parade I was leading—because rain was still falling everywhere else in Atlanta, but not here. We began to ride, and it felt almost as if my bike were pedaling itself.

At twenty-eight miles, we reached our turnaround point. Elizabeth stood there beside a cooler filled with sushi, Monster energy drinks, salt-and-vinegar potato chips—everything I'd had requested.

"This is the best bike ride ever," I told her. "Do me a favor and call Sunny and tell her to get her butt over here and ride with me. I don't want her to miss this."

There's a phrase that triathletes often use, "Don't get too high, don't get too low." An athlete who allows himself to take excessive joy from a tailwind is likely to be crushed by the next headwind. All racers discover sooner or later how important it is to control their emotions during a long race, not to allow their mental state to become dependent on how things are going. It's easy enough to learn this lesson, but much harder to practice it, especially when you're pushing your body and mind beyond known limits. For two straight days, things had gone mostly my way, and I was riding high, maybe too high.

When I completed the first lap, all my cycling companions quit, leaving me friendless for lap two. (Sunny was unable to join me because Jordan had stranded her without a vehicle at Jason's home 40 minutes away.) I found Jason under one of three pop-up tents that had been set up at the staging area.

"Find a bike," I told him. "You're riding with me."

As we pedaled along together, Jason, riding a machine he'd borrowed from Elizabeth, we chatted about this and that and eventually landed on the subject of golf, a shared passion. Over the past twenty-one days, golf had become for me a potent symbol of leisure and escape. More than any other topic of conversation, it took my mind away from hip pain, saddle sores and sleepiness, making six hours of turning the pedals pass by a little less tediously. Jason mentioned that he had seen the Masters tournament at nearby Augusta National Golf Club a few times.

"Man, I'd love to do that," I said.

"I'll tell you what," Jason said. "If you finish this thing, I'll take you with me next year. But only if you finish."

"I'm going to hold you to that," I said.

At the turnaround point, I paused for a while to ice my knees, which had swollen to the size of softballs. On the way back, a woman wearing a North Georgia Triathlon Club kit and riding a Specialized Crux cyclo-cross bike came cruising toward us, pulled a 180, and fell in beside us. She was obviously a friend of Jason's.

"How do I make myself useful?" she asked.

"You can take a turn pulling," Jason said.

I struck up a conversation with the newcomer. She seemed interested in me and my journey, but she didn't ask the kinds of questions many supporters asked when they first met me. I thought nothing of it until Jason spoke up.

"You have no idea who you're talking to, do you?" he asked.

"No, I don't," I said cautiously. "Should I?"

"That's Renee!" he said.

"Renee, Renee," I said, trying to think.

"The massage therapist you were just raving to me about!" Jason said, cackling in amazement.

My jaw fell open. I remembered perfectly well the fantastic pre- and post-swim massages this woman had given me, but I couldn't have picked her out of a police lineup.

"Don't take it personally," I said. "I don't fully wake up until I'm on my bike." (If then.)

The nearest thing to adversity I faced during the remainder of the ride was a light drizzle. When we finished, Jason returned Elizabeth's bike to her and then waved me toward him.

"Come here," he said. "I've got something for you."

He led me a short distance to a splash pad that a handful of children were capering around on. My ambassador joined right in, hurdling through waterspouts and flapping his arms like a six-year-old. I marched straight to the gushing center geyser and stood in it, allowing the refreshing water to jet upward over my body. The film crew had followed us, and with the camera rolling, I hammed up my expression of carnal ecstasy. I had experienced more comforts in the last thirty-six hours than I had in the preceding three weeks. There was the relaxing soak in Santa Rosa Sound with my kids, the renewed strength of my body, Dallas and Kyle's rejoining the campaign, the excellence of the Silver Comet Trail, Renee's massages, and now this impromptu hydro-massage. What next?

The marathon went according to script. Sixty people ran the 5K and then went home. I ran on in the dark with Jason, Elizabeth, and a few others. Renee joined us at mile thirteen, and I was quite pleased with myself for recognizing her, despite the darkness and her switch to running clothes. At ten o'clock, we stopped at the staging area so I could kiss Sunny's lips and my children's heads before they rolled out for South Carolina. Two hours later, triathlon number twenty-two was in the books.

"I could eat a horse," I told Jason, whom I had astonished a few hours earlier by wolfing down a heaping plate of ribs, macaroni and cheese, and salad during a ten-minute break from running.

"I've got something better," Jason said.

He disappeared momentarily and came back with a stack of Styrofoam containers, smiling like he had *Christmas* presents for all of us to enjoy. I opened a box and found a row of hot, fresh chicken enchiladas from Costa Vida, my favorite restaurant chain. My friend Dano, who owns several Costa Vida franchises, had arranged this treat from afar.

Without warning, I felt a powerful upwelling of tearful sentimentality and swallowed it back with some difficulty. In the perpetually raw emotional state the Fifty had put me in, those enchiladas seemed to me more than enchiladas—they were a sign that someone was looking out for me, that everything would be okay.

To conserve time, I ate in the back of the van on the way to the home of a supporter, Chip, who lived close by and had volunteered the use of his shower. Renee gave me one last massage on the way. The pleasure of the flavors on my tongue and of the practiced fingers on my flesh, layered atop all the other tailwinds of the past two days, made me feel as relaxed and contented as if I were walking a lush, green fairway after hitting a perfect drive.

Don't get too high.

We pulled up in front of a row of townhomes just off the freeway and Chip led us into his unit. His wife, eight months pregnant, was woken by our boisterous entrance. She came down to greet us, looking less than thrilled. I couldn't blame her.

5 DON'T GET TOO HIGH

A bunch of smelly strangers had just burst into her home unexpectedly at midnight, and her belly looked about ready to pop.

Chip seemed—or pretended—not to notice his wife's exhausted expression and played the perfect host, supplying bananas, protein shakes, and other refreshments. I got first dibs on the shower, then waited in Chip's man cave while Dallas and Kyle took their turns. It was my kind of room, outfitted with a large flat-screen TV and an Xbox and used to store several thousand dollars' worth of bikes. Chip's wife wanted to turn it into a nursery.

"Good luck winning that battle," I teased him.

Soon it was time for final farewells. I thanked Jason sincerely for all he had done to make the day a success.

"I'll see you back here next spring for the Masters," he said.

"Darn right you will!" I said.

I felt as sure as I sounded. At last, I had turned a corner, both geographically (we were no longer moving east) and metaphorically. The worst of my trials were behind me. Florida and Georgia represented a new beginning, a blueprint for the second half of the campaign. All I had to do now was recreate the past two days for the next twenty-eight, and I would practically coast to the final finish line.

I was fooling myself.

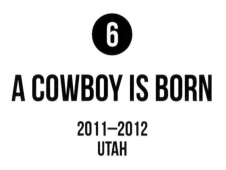

A COWBOY IS BORN

2011–2012
UTAH

Soon after I set my first world record, I began to plot the next one, registering for thirty iron-distance triathlons taking place in the 2012 season. No athlete had ever completed more than twenty such events in a calendar year. I had still done only one—ever. Figuring a little more practice couldn't hurt, I planned a dress rehearsal at Ironman Canada in August 2011.

My friend Tyrell, who happened to be a real cowboy, signed up for the race as well and talked me into joining him in wearing a cowboy hat during the marathon, but at the last minute, he backed out, citing lack of preparation. My family insisted I wear the hat anyway, so that they could see me easily amongst the other racers. In retrospect, I'm glad I did. What I had expected to be a cause of embarrassment turned out to be a huge hit among spectators. I heard more than a few shouts of "Go, cowboy!" as I paced through the streets of Penticton, British Columbia. Sunny, who stood among those spectators, appreciated the hat and was excited that I complied with her request.

After hearing people around her call me 'The Cowboy' during the event, she said to me afterward, "That's it! The Iron Cowboy!"

"Me? A cowboy?" I laughed. "That's a joke. I'm allergic to horses . . . and hay."

Sunny and I later discussed this idea as a real idea, and the more we thought about it, the more excited we got. *The Iron Cowboy* was such a cool name, and an actual title that I could use during this world record. Wearing the cowboy hat was the perfect way for me to stand out in races, allowing people to identify me and join the fundraising for the charity, In Our Own Quiet Way. It later became a creative way to include my family, being that my kids would pick out the hats for me. These hats ranged from pink with sequin to tiger print, never a dull moment in my cowboy hat. I wore them proudly as I raced, feeling my family's presence.

Complicating my preparations for the iron-distance triathlon world record was my family's still-dire financial situation. Days after we returned home from Penticton, foreclosure on our home became real, and we were kicked out. My father-in-law, who was now on *his* way toward bankruptcy, bailed us out yet again by allowing us to move into a rental house he owned that was also in foreclosure.

Twenty-five hours a week of training left me with little time to pursue gainful employment. My sole source of income was triathlon coaching, which brought in a meager income. Sunny earned what she could through "emotional work," as she called it, and babysat as well. Together this only totaled around a thousand bucks a month. Friends helped us in a variety of ways. Those with gardens brought over vegetables in the summer, laundry detergent was doorbell ditched at our door, even an anonymous Sub for Santa brought all our kids' Christmas presents that year.

The biggest and most worrisome expense looming over me was airfare. I planned to race in eleven countries on four continents. My blood pressure dropped a good ten points when ASEA, a supplements brand that had sponsored my first record attempt, stepped up to pay for all my flights, foreign and domestic. Around the same time, the CEO of BioStructures (a medical device company), a guy named Russell, agreed to buy me a bike on the condition that I sign it and hand it over to him after race number thirty. Russell's confidence that I would actually make it that far meant almost as much to me as the $10,000 Specialized Shiv I purchased with his money.

When a man visits four continents and eleven countries in one year—even if it's not for the sake of doing 140.6-mile triathlons—some things are bound to go wrong. In March, I flew all the way to New Zealand to do what was to be my third race of the year. At a meeting held the day before the event was scheduled to take place, I learned that, due to forecasted high winds, it had been downgraded to a half-iron-distance event. I did it anyway, then flew back home, and two weeks later turned around and flew to Melbourne, Australia, to take a second crack at my third iron-distance triathlon. All told, I spent eighty-four hours traveling to two islands, located two hours apart, when only one of those events would count toward my record attempt.

Some things went wrong on the racecourse too. My sixth event took place in

❻ A COWBOY IS BORN

Marble Falls, Texas. I traveled there after spending one day at home, following a for-ty-one-hour return trip from Ironman South Africa. I had an unusually good swim and left the water in twelfth place. Thirty miles into the bike course, I took over the lead. The motorcycle escort that came with the lead made me feel like a super-star, and I began to push even harder—too hard, given the 95-degree weather. At one hundred miles, my right leg cramped so badly I had to complete the remaining twelve miles using only my left leg.

My unraveling continued in the marathon. At mile five, I was forced to slow from a jog to a walk to get my heart rate under control. Three miles later, I threw up every ounce of liquid I had swallowed in the preceding six hours. I then began to hear a strange buzzing in my left ear. At mile seventeen, my entire body suddenly went into full rigor, and I toppled to the ground like dead wood. Tyrell had come to the race to support me, and he witnessed my collapse. Panicked, he threw me into the back of his pickup truck and rushed to the transition area, where I received a saline IV.

As I lay on the ground with the tube in my arm, Tyrell's phone rang. He spoke a few words and then tried to hand the device to me.

"It's Sunny," he said.

"Not now," I told him. "I need some time."

Five minutes later, Tyrell got a second call. This time it was Lucy, who was nine years old. *No fair.* I took the phone.

"What's wrong, Daddy?" she asked. "Are you okay?"

"My legs won't work, Lucy," I said. "I had to stop."

"But can't you just walk the rest of the way?"

"I don't think so," I said.

"Can you crawl?" Lucy asked.

I began to cry.

"It's too far to crawl," I croaked.

"Can you cartwheel?"

I laughed through my tears.

"I'll try, sweetie," I said.

When I hung up, I asked Tyrell to fetch Mark, the race director. Typically, when a competitor hitches a ride in the back of a pickup truck, he is disqualified, but I asked Mark to make an exception for me, and he granted it. So I got back into Tyrell's truck, and he returned me to the spot where I had collapsed. From there, I walked all but the very last step of the nine miles remaining in my sixth iron-distance triathlon of 2012—and then I cartwheeled across the finish line.

A week later, I was in St. George, Utah, where Sunny was to make her Ironman debut at my side. She had been waking up as early as one-thirty a.m. to squeeze in her training, and running back-and-forth in front of the house so that our young children could call to her if they needed her. She had crafted a frilly pink tutu to wear during the marathon and had decorated my cowboy hat to match with some of the same material.

Half a mile into the swim, a sudden and violent wind squall struck, turning the lake into a blender. The big orange buoys marking the course disappeared behind walls of water. I heard screams all around me. Safety kayaks capsized, and swimmers clung to them like shipwrecked sailors. One by one, the buoys broke loose and floated away. I set my sights instead on a giant rock that marked the turnaround point. Sunny remained calm, but her progress through the bludgeoning surf as a beginner swimmer was slow, and I became concerned about the clock. I checked my watch and saw we'd been swimming for an hour and forty minutes, leaving us just forty minutes to make the cutoff. I asked Sunny if she felt safe, and if it was okay for me to swim ahead.

"Go get 'em Cowboy!" she said as she cheerfully fought through the waves.

I reached the shore with just over a two-hours swim time and then waited on the ramp for Sunny. She staggered out of the reservoir twenty minutes later, two minutes past the cut-off, crying, barely able to stand. She was exhausted after swimming for two hours and twenty-two minutes, with a heart rate over 180. The race officials allowed her to continue, but requested her timing chip, not accepting it as an official Ironman finish. She slipped past them before they took the timing chip and rushed into transition. She cried from fatigue and tried to get her things together to start the bike.

We mounted our bikes and headed out into 40 mph headwinds. Sunny was still trying to recover nutritionally from the swim and struggled to maintain a pace that would enable us to make the next cutoff at the end of the bike leg. I kept drifting ahead, hoping to pull her along with me (without actually giving her an illegal draft), then drifting back to her when I saw that she just couldn't ride any faster. At mile thirty, Sunny blew a tire, the first flat of her bike riding history. She called out to me, but the wind swallowed her voice, and I rode on without being aware of her crisis. I was more than a mile down the road when I realized I'd lost her. I pulled over and dismounted to wait, but after several minutes she still hadn't appeared, so I clipped in and rode back the way I'd come, drawing odd looks from other racers. When I came upon Sunny, she had just finished fixing her tire.

We were approaching mile forty when a race official drew alongside us on a scooter. I asked him about the bike time cutoff, and he informed us there was an intermediate cutoff point at mile sixty-four. I did some math in my head and realized I would have to ride as hard as I could for the next twenty-four miles to have any chance of making it, and that Sunny had no chance. I turned to her.

"Just go," she said, deflated.

I made the cutoff by one minute, but my regret vastly outweighed my relief for how awfully the day had turned out for Sunny. When I reached my spot in the transition area, I found that her tutu had been stuffed into my transition bag. I put it on, feeling a deep sense of connection with my wife, had my matching cowboy hat, and ran the marathon. I was now symbolically completing the race for Sunny while also giving everyone a measure of humor to enjoy as they spectated.

In late June, I flew to Germany to begin an extended European leg of my quest. I would race five Ironmans in five weeks, in five countries (including a quick jaunt back to the States for Ironman Coeur d'Alene). My bank account was out of money; I had $10 left. Out of the blue, my friend Vicki from Canada messaged me on Facebook, asking how she could help (knowing I would never dare ask). I mentioned that I was out of money, and if I could come up with enough to cover the car rental, it would double as a place to sleep. She and her boyfriend Jihad surprised me and deposited $400 into my account. I now had money for the rental car, and could maybe squeeze some change out of that to cover some food while traveling. There would be times in the weeks ahead when I would resort to making meals out of free energy bar samples given out at race expos, just so that I could afford to put gas in my rental car.

Hotels were completely out of the question, and just three days before my departure for Munich, my first homestay fell through. An urgent Facebook plea led to an invitation from an older couple who lived forty-five miles away from Regensburg, site of triathlon number eleven. This couple picked me up at the airport, fed me unfamiliar foods (white asparagus, intentionally undercooked eggs), took me on walking and cycling tours of local attractions (including Regensburg Cathedral and the most impressive farmer's market I've ever seen). All in all, they gave me a Bavarian experience that I had never had, and would never forget. It was this kind of experience that was special, and that I would have never experienced if I'd had money to spend. This pattern continued for my whole stint in Europe.

A Swedish woman named Szilvia, a friend of a friend from church, for reasons I will never know, made heroic efforts to hook me up with hosts in each country. She found me Alice in Klagenfurt, who fed me a delicious chicken Alfredo. Then Daniele in Italy, who reacted with horror when I took away leftover pizza from a restaurant to eat cold the next day. Also, Isabelle and Jerome in Perpignan, who let me into their home two hours after learning of my existence from Szilvia. In Zurich, I stayed with Tony and Julienna, a beautiful interracial couple whose three-year-old boy called me Jason all week.

Swimming, cycling, and running were a relatively small part of the overall experience. In a typical week, I did no exercise whatsoever on Monday, Tuesday, Wednesday, and Saturday. On Thursday, travel permitting, I rode my bike nice and easy to loosen up the old legs. On Friday, I did a short swim and a bike ride at the race site to get a feel for the course. Then on Sunday, I swam, biked, and ran 140.6 miles as fast as I could. In my abundant free time, I did touristy stuff like watching a mountain stage of the Tour de France in person and visiting the Palais des Papes (the Popes' Palace) in Avignon. Record or no record, I was living a life that beat the heck out of spending sixty hours a week selling mortgages. In the blink of an eye, it was over.

On the morning of July 17, I found myself at the Air France check-in counter at Kloten Airport in Zurich with a big problem. Having spent most of my remaining funds on small gifts for Sunny and the kids, I lacked the money I needed to check my bike for the flight to New York. The customer service agent wanted 220 euros. I explained to her in broken French that I had only 105 euros left on my cash card, and I begged her to take it and waive the balance. She held firm.

I sweetened my offer by pulling a ten-euro note from my pocket and placing it on the counter next to the cash card. The agent shook her head. I fished in my pockets again and came up with a bunch of coins. Another head shake. I found fifty-eight American dollars and added them to the pile. She directed me to a currency exchange kiosk. I went there, traded my dollars for Euros, and brought them to the agent. My flight was due to begin boarding in thirty minutes. The woman told me I was still eighty-five euros short.

"Please," I said, and then just walked away, leaving the bike with her, not yet officially checked.

I slept not one second during the entire transatlantic flight, fretting about how I would explain the loss of the bike to Russell from BioStructures—and about what

⑥ A COWBOY IS BORN

the heck I was going to ride at Ironman Lake Placid. When I recognized my well-used bike case, as it appeared in the baggage claim, I nearly wept with relief. The only hitch was that I now couldn't afford to check the bike for my flight to Lake Placid, so I left it with a friend who lived in Manhattan and arranged to do my next race on a borrowed bike.

The evening before that race, I called Sunny from my host's home to catch up on the news about my family, whom I hadn't seen in more than a month and missed viscerally like an inmate misses decent food. The news was that our one remaining family car had been repossessed the previous night. This one wasn't my fault—a bank error was to blame—but it made no practical difference. For the next eight months, Sunny would be forced to get around on a 90cc scooter that one of my athlete clients traded me in place of cash; fortunately, her sister Shauna lent us an old van to use until we could afford to purchase a car.

Race number twenty-seven took place in Lake Havasu, Arizona. By that point I had already broken the record—now I was just padding my stats. I started the race wearing the usual gear (wetsuit, swim cap, and goggles) plus one extra item: a fiberglass cord wrapped around my waist and trailing back to an inflated raft with a fifteen-year-old-boy inside.

I had learned about Dayton, who has cerebral palsy, from a viral YouTube video titled *Dayton's Legs*. The story is of Dayton's friendship with a boy his age named Spencer, who, by his own initiative, had done a short triathlon with Dayton. He pulled him through the water in a raft, towing him over the bike course in a trailer, and pushing him to the finish line in a contraption similar to a baby jogger. As a teenager, I had worked with physically challenged kids, and I remembered well how much joy they took in going bowling and doing other fun stuff they couldn't do without some assistance—and how satisfying it was for me to provide such assistance. So I reached out to Dayton's mother, Sherrine, and asked her if her son would like to become an Ironman.

Dayton communicates with his eyes. A blink means *yes,* a stare means *no.* Sherrine put my question to him. He blinked and blinked and blinked.

I had expected it would be difficult to drag a seventy-one pound human for 2.4 miles in a lake, but it turned out to be relatively easy. The key, I discovered, was to maintain a completely steady tempo, as any slackening of the rope between us required me to rebuild our momentum from zero. Our official time for the first leg of the race was a respectable eighty minutes.

IRON COWBOY

The trouble began when I rolled out of the transition area on my bike, with Dayton seated behind me in his trailer. From the very first pedal stroke, I felt the trailer yawing to the left, creating a braking effect. It was a bit like pushing a shopping cart with a wonky wheel. I knew that some simple adjustment could probably correct the issue, but I was more confident in my fitness than in my mechanical skills, so I decided to muscle my way through it.

Over the first nine miles, the unexpected technical glitch did nothing worse than annoy me. Then we came to a giant hill. Dayton's trailer weighed almost as much as he did. By the time I reached the top of the climb, my thighs were shattered. I still had one hundred miles left to cover, and I would have to ascend the same hill three more times in two directions.

In the previous weekend's race in Florida, I had completed the bike leg in five hours and nine minutes, but in Lake Havasu, it took me the same amount of time to complete the first *half* of the bike route. We were averaging eleven miles per hour and had no hope whatsoever of making the bike cutoff time. When I looked back at Dayton, I saw he had slumped over to the right side of his trailer with an unfocused look in his eyes. He wasn't having any more fun than I was.

Sunny knew that I had been biking much longer than I had expected and that I would need calories, so she picked up a Double-Double, a large order of French fries, and a strawberry shake from In-N-Out Burger. She also had her bike and was ready to ride with me. Unfortunately, neither the replenished calories, nor Sunny's company, helped me ride any faster as we started the second lap. An authentic Jedi of positive thinking, Sunny tried everything she could think of to motivate me and lift Dayton's spirits, but to no avail.

She prayed and prayed, pleading for a solution to alleviate my burdens. Riding just behind us on our left side, Sunny reached out to lay a hand on Dayton's trailer as she made her plea to God. The moment her fingers touched the frame, the trailer straightened out and the wonky wheel feeling vanished.

"Sunny!" I shouted. "Keep your hand there!"

This wasn't quite the miracle Sunny had been expecting, but it seemed to be an answer to her plea. Riding with one hand on her aero bar pad and the other on Dayton's trailer was as challenging for her as pulling Dayton was for me, but her sacrifice made a crucial difference on the big hill. Our average speed increased, and I was able to preserve just enough strength in my legs to contemplate running a marathon.

The sun went down. Technically, that meant our race was over, as athletes are required to carry their own lighting after dark, and we hadn't planned on being out this long, but a security officer took pity on us and lighted our way back to the transition area with his high beams. We got there three hours and thirteen minutes after the cutoff time had come and gone; however, more than five hours remained before the final race cutoff at midnight. I found the race director, Mark—the same guy who had allowed me to complete my "cartwheel" race in Marble Falls—and begged him to let us continue.

"I can make the last cutoff," I said. "Let me run."

Mark looked from me to Dayton and back to me again, then agreed. Dayton's father, Wes, transferred him to his running chair and we were off. Sherrine and my friend Ashley ran with us. All was well until we came to London Bridge—the real thing, which Lake Havasu had bought from the Brits and relocated piece by piece in the late 1960s—at which point we had to execute a kind of portage. I lifted Dayton up and over while Wes carried his chair. The marathon course crossed this point six times.

At 11:36 p.m., twenty-four minutes before the final cutoff time, Lucy and Lily—up way past their bedtimes—joined us for the stretch run toward the finish line. I got so fired up that I began to sprint, and my daughters struggled to keep up. Within yards of the finish line, we transitioned from a paved path to soft grass. The wheels of Dayton's chair sunk in, and suddenly I felt as though I were back on that killer hill on the bike course. It seemed a fitting way for the day to end. I walked Dayton in from there as the very few surviving spectators—Sunny, Mark, our friend Brittany, and a couple of others—made the noise of a much larger crowd. My exhaustion was absolute, but my satisfaction was even greater. Placing the finisher's medal around Dayton's neck felt better than receiving my own finisher's medal ever had.

The next morning, our family piled into a Chevy Suburban that had been loaned to me by my friend Jacques (we still had no vehicle of our own) for a four-hour drive to Phoenix, site of my next race. I did a lot of thinking along the way. Strangely, I found myself in the same dissatisfied, hungry state of mind after completing my twenty-seventh iron-distance triathlon of 2012 that I'd been in after finishing my twenty-second half-iron-distance triathlon of 2010. My second world record had done little more than the first to solve Africa's water crisis or to restore solvency to the Lawrence household.

These disappointments did not cause me to second-guess my choice to go down the path of endurance pioneering, rather they made me want to go further. I still believed in the journey; I just hadn't completed it.

But there was another reason to go further. As challenging as the past year had been, it had not pushed me to my limit, physically or mentally. I now recognized the deeper purpose of this lengthy journey that I had embarked on, beginning in 2010. It was to discover the ultimate limit of my physical and mental endurance—and perhaps of human endurance. That's a heck of a thing to sign up for, but it felt right to me, a mission I had been put on this earth to carry out.

All these thoughts had been swirling around in my mind for some time, but my experience with Dayton had given them a new dimension. It struck me that there was a little Dayton in everyone, including me. A boy with cerebral palsy can't have what society would consider a normal life, and he most certainly can't do an Ironman—except if he believes he can. An unemployed beginner triathlete can't make a new career out of setting triathlon world records—unless he takes the first step anyway, and keeps on taking the next step. At some point in life, every person dreams of doing something that seems impossible. For the most part, each of us is on our own to discover that it is possible if we only believe and we just don't quit.

We're not entirely on our own, because we can draw inspiration to achieve our own impossible, by seeing others conquer theirs. This effect is never more powerful than when the most ordinary people do the most extraordinary things. When I began my endurance journey, I wasn't sure how this journey would affect the charity, my family or me. But crossing that finish line with Dayton had opened my mind. The purpose of continuing my journey was not only to self-actualize, to feed my family, and to raise money for a good cause, but to help others achieve their dreams, whatever they might be.

Completing this mission would require something truly outlandish—not a small step but a giant leap. My final challenge—the goal that, if I achieved it, would redefine human limits—would have to be one that seemed utterly impossible to absolutely everyone.

"I have an idea," I said to Sunny somewhere around the town of Buckeye.

She looked at me nervously, knowing that this phrase was always a dangerous introduction, "Oh no..." she said in a quiet voice.

"What if I did an iron-distance triathlon—not an official one but my own thing—in all fifty states, in fifty consecutive days?"

Sunny dropped her head in disbelief.

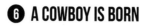 6 A COWBOY IS BORN

ANOTHER DAY, ANOTHER DIAGNOSIS

DAYS 23–24
SOUTH CAROLINA, NORTH CAROLINA

At six forty-five in the morning on Day 23, I staggered bleary-eyed onto a sun-bleached concrete outdoor pool deck at the Waterbridge residential community in Myrtle Beach, South Carolina. At the opposite end of the pool stood fifty-plus members of the Myrtle Beach Triathlon Club clad in racing attire. Addressing them through a PA system was the club's vice president, Michael, his amplified baritone delivering rules and safety guidelines for a sprint competition that would begin shortly in the same pool that I was about to use for my daily 2.4 miles. Seeing me emerge from the men's changing room, Michael paused his speech to acknowledge my presence.

"The Iron Cowboy is with us this morning," he said, like a bandleader introducing his trombonist.

There was a light applause and some cheering. I waved.

"Keep the dream alive," Michael added. "How are you holding up?"

I forced a smile and held up a thumb, hoping these gestures would exhaust the natives' curiosity. Not so. Michael and the others now waited expectantly for me to jump in the water. The problem was that I was physically incapable of doing so. The muscles on my inner thighs that had cramped four days before in Mississippi were still tender and would cramp again at the slightest provocation. Any form of leaping action was out of the question. Swallowing my dignity, I entered the pool in the only way I could, by passively keeling over like an axed tree, flopping onto my side and making a big splash. My audience guffawed, assuming I was trying to be funny.

IRON COWBOY

For whatever reason, almost every adult member of our party—Casey, Aaron, Kyle, and Sunny—decided this would be the day they'd all swim with me. They quickly lost interest in turning laps, however, and transitioned to horsing around, making thongs out of their swimsuits by stuffing the fabric between their butt cheeks and then executing a succession of dolphin dives, piercing the surface with their mostly bare bottoms each time. I was too tired to be amused.

By the time I had completed my swim, eaten breakfast, and changed into my cycling gear, the locals had finished their entire triathlon. One of them, eight-year-old Cameron, was accorded the honor of leading me to the community's front gate and onto my bike route astride a Day-Glo BMX bike, his head protected by a helmet decorated with a Mohawk of rubber spikes.

"Take it slow," I half joked. "I'm an old man."

A handful of adults continued with me after Cameron stopped. A support and gear (or SAG) vehicle, piloted by Elizabeth, another Myrtle Beach Triathlon Club member, trailing behind us. Every twenty miles or so, she pulled over to the shoulder ahead of us and handed us drinks, snacks, and cold sponges. At the halfway point, we paused at the Claire Chapin Epps Family YMCA, where a few of my companions bailed out, and some others joined. Among the newcomers was Adam, who had participated in the earlier sprint triathlon. As we nibbled away at the second half of the ride, Adam began to tell me his story.

"I used to weigh 320 pounds," he said. (I heard a lot of stories that started this way.) "Not that long ago, in fact. Then I just got tired of being a fat guy."

Adam bought a bike and started riding. When the weather got too cold to ride, he switched to running. When it got too cold to run, he switched to swimming indoors. Without intending to, he'd become a triathlete. The following summer, he signed up for a sprint triathlon, and then another, and another. The pounds melted off, a process that was helped along by sensible dietary changes such as replacing forty daily ounces of Coke with an equal volume of water.

Adam had lost sixty-five pounds so far. His two children had done this morning's triathlon with him, and his wife had started running. His pride was unmistakable.

"I'll tell you what, though," he concluded. "The thought of doing just one Ironman still scares the heck out of me."

"Do you think I wasn't scared when I got in the pool this morning?" I asked. "Seriously, though: if you really want to, you'll get there someday."

❼ ANOTHER DAY, ANOTHER DIAGNOSIS

The video crew was again with us. They did some filming on the move from the back of an SUV that they had rented, and they also stopped periodically to fire up a drone and capture aerial footage. At one point, Jared, who was operating the drone, flew it too close to a power line, which somehow interfered with the signal from the remote control. Suddenly the drone plummeted toward earth like a falcon dive-bombing a field mouse. It was less than ten feet from impact when the signal reconnected, and Jared got it to level off. The drone was now flying straight at Adam's head, but he ducked just in time to avoid having an ear taken off. The reading on his heart rate monitor jumped instantly from 120 beats per minute to 170.

Around eighty miles, a tight spot formed on the back of my left knee. Over the next hour, it became increasingly uncomfortable. I pictured a boil swelling on my hamstring tendon. By one hundred miles it felt as though it were about to burst, spewing puss onto the rider behind me. I paused my pedaling and tried to contort my body in such a way that I could peek at the crook of my knee, where I expected to find an angry red welt. All that I discovered was that it is physically impossible to see the crook of your knee when you're riding a bike.

As we headed back toward the YMCA, Elizabeth pulled up next to us in the SAG vehicle.

"Pete's going to get you some dinner," she said, referring to the Myrtle Beach Triathlon Club president. "Any requests?"

"I want a porterhouse steak, cooked medium well, garlic mashed potatoes, and steamed vegetables," I said.

Before the campaign had started, David had told me that if I ever craved something specific, I should go ahead and eat it, because my body would be in survival mode and it would know what it needed. Back in Calgary, I used to order the porterhouse steak with garlic mashed potatoes at my favorite restaurant, the Keg, and I had a nostalgic craving for that meal now.

When we returned to the YMCA, the food was waiting, enough for everyone. I gobbled mine while lying on a table and getting worked on by Carla, a massage therapist who'd come all the way from Hilton Head to help out. I told Dallas about the pain behind my left knee, and he ran the cold laser over it. I thought about asking him what he thought it was, but I held back, afraid of what I might hear.

The video guys did some more filming during the Iron Cowboy 5K, which had about twenty participants. Jared was waiting near our turnaround point, remote control in hand. The drone buzzed high overhead. Jared attempted a flyover, but he botched it, catching a propeller on a high branch of a big old oak tree. The sound—similar to that of a Weedwacker hitting a boulder—caught everyone's attention.

Time slowed as the drone entered freefall. Jared's eyes bugged out, and in the next instant, he dashed toward the spot where his $1,500 toy was potentially landing. He was willing to lay out for it like a wide receiver diving for an overthrown football if necessary, but at the very last moment he seemed to recognize the high probability that the accelerating hunk of metal would kill him, and he pulled up. The drone smashed into the pavement with a cringe-inducing racket and shattered into several pieces. The runner it came closest to pulverizing was—who else?—Adam.

"Ha!" he crowed. "Karma!"

Elizabeth continued to trail behind me in her vehicle as I ground out the rest of the marathon with five supporters. We hadn't gone far when I waved her forward.

"You wouldn't happen to have any toilet paper in there, would you?" I asked.

"As a matter of fact, I do," she said.

Elizabeth reached into the back seat and produced a fresh roll, then handed it to me through the window. We were passing through a swampy area. I picked my way through it in search of a discreet place to answer nature's call. Back on the road, Elizabeth suddenly remembered that alligators were rumored to inhabit the swamp, but it was too late to warn me. Of all the ways in which my quest might have ended prematurely, being eaten by an alligator while I was relieving myself would probably have been the most inglorious.

I finished running at eleven fifteen. One of my five surviving supporters, Gage, looked at his watch and wondered out loud how he was ever going to get through a busy Monday at work the next day.

"Yeah, you've got it pretty rough," I said.

"Touché."

I climbed into the motor home with some difficulty, my left knee having stiffened into a rheumatic ball of pain after I stopped moving. Casey took the wheel and drove to the Island Vista Resort, a magnificent beachfront property where Elizabeth had booked a room for my family and crew to use as a home base for the day. We took an elevator to the top floor, and Aaron led us into a three-bedroom ocean-view suite. It was one of the more opulent hotel rooms I had ever entered. All the beds were unmade. I pictured my crew luxuriating between those soft sheets while I was outdoors in the blistering heat, suffering through 140.6 human-powered miles, and a wave of raw envy swept over me. Yet, I was grateful that my kids had somewhere

❼ ANOTHER DAY, ANOTHER DIAGNOSIS

incredible to spend their day.

Dallas gave my new injury some more attention on the drive north to Charlotte. As he did, my thoughts turned to Tim, my first American friend, who had helped me survive missionary training in 1995 and with whom I had lived briefly in 1999 when I moved to Utah. Although we eventually drifted apart, Tim remained an important figure in my life. After all, if he hadn't welcomed my visit I'd funded with my Ferris wheel winnings, I might never have met Sunny or become the Iron Cowboy.

Like me, Tim had married young and fathered five children. Less than a year before I started my campaign, Tim took his kids to a park to play. He lay down under a tree, fell asleep, and never woke up. Dead at thirty-seven. Blood clot. His passing had left me with a somewhat irrational fear of suffering the same fate. I knew I could gut my way through shoulder pain, and that even the worst blister would heal if properly treated. A blood clot, however, could take me out like a lightning strike.

The pain I was experiencing now in the crook of my left knee—a pain so concentrated that even the slightest pressure from Dallas's hands caused a reflexive twitch of the leg—was different from any I had ever known. I wondered if I would recognize the feeling of a blood clot...

I was deep asleep in the RV at four o'clock the next morning when Casey dropped Kyle and Dallas at Charlotte Douglas International Airport for an early flight back to Utah to catch up on their lives at home before rejoining the campaign later. I was still asleep forty-five minutes later when Casey parked the RV at the home of Izzy, my North Carolina ambassador, on Lake Norman. At six o'clock, when I was supposed to start swimming, I was still sleeping. Still snoring at six forty-five, Casey and Aaron, having been rebuffed in their first few attempts to rouse me, returned to my bedside with an ultimatum.

"There's a girl out there who came to sing the national anthem for you," Aaron said. "She has to leave for summer camp in a few minutes. It's now or never, bud."

The thought of disappointing a child was at that moment just about the only thing that seemed more unbearable to me than swimming—and Aaron knew it. I got up and dressed in a wrinkled T-shirt and saggy shorts. My new injury had knotted up even more overnight, and my first steps were torturous. Casey took one elbow, Aaron the other, and I hobbled gingerly down a long driveway toward Izzy's large, seven-figure crib. When I came around the side of the house, I yawned, rubbed my eyes, and saw a wedding-size group of people gathered dockside at the far end of a lush lawn, bathed in yolky morning light. Everyone looked so . . . awake.

Having seen my visit as an opportunity to unite the large and vibrant—but somewhat fractured—endurance community in Charlotte, Izzy had reached out to all the local swim, bike, run, and triathlon clubs and invited them to collaborate in hosting me. He'd held weekly conference calls with the various team leaders. Izzy had searched for and found a corporate partner to underwrite the day's expenses. He'd created a Facebook page and commemorative T-shirts, which many in the crowd were now wearing. In short, Izzy had busted his butt to make this day special, and as my eyes took in the first evidence that it would be, my heart swelled with gratitude.

Things looked rather different from the perspective of the fifty-plus people who watched me wobble toward them between steadying hands. The impression I made with my broken-man entrance was one that frightened everyone there. I saw the same disillusioned look on every face—a look that said, *There is absolutely no way this guy can possibly do an Ironman triathlon today.*

Izzy stepped forward and introduced me, then handed me a microphone. Immediately, my throat constricted and my vision swam. Several long seconds passed before I could utter a single word.

"I've been looking forward to North Carolina for a long time," I said quietly. "There were days when I thought I would never get here. But I knew how hard you were working for me, and I kept telling myself, *You can't let them down.*" I paused to collect myself. "Thank you for giving me something to hope for." That was all I could manage. I passed the mic back to Izzy, who gave it to Haley, our anthem singer. I looked around and saw glassy eyes everywhere. At that moment, everyone there was filled with empathy, each person feeling my gratitude, and also the effort it took to get to North Carolina.

Twenty minutes later, my now permanently distended stomach filled with egg casserole and hash browns, I was in the water. Izzy had enlisted a pair of top local swimmers—both named Heather—to serve as my swim guides. He had even taken the trouble to measure out a buoy-marked course that I was to circumnavigate three times to achieve the required distance. While I thrashed along in the two Heathers' slipstream, Casey got sucked into an impromptu race with a strong high school swimmer. On the last lap, Casey surged ahead. He swam right up to the shore and continued to flail away as if unaware he had beached himself, provoking laughter from the spectators. Then he stood and raised his arms overhead à la Rocky Balboa. "South Carolina!" he shouted. "This is awesome!"

The laughter stopped, and an awkward silence took its place.

"North Carolina," someone corrected.

It was bound to happen sooner or later.

I was well into my own final lap when I realized that I was again going to hit 2.4 miles before I reached shore. The moment it happened, I grabbed hold of a nearby kayak and asked its surprised operator to tow me to Izzy's dock. I flipped onto my back and glided with my eyes closed, the sun warming my face. It was peaceful, and so relaxing, to forget everything for just a few seconds, gazing into the sky as I floated on my back.

A gentle impact startled me.

"Were you *asleep?*" the kayaker asked, looking down at me.

Back on land, I chowed more egg casserole and hash browns while Rob, a local doctor, attempted to draw my blood—another health check. My resting heart rate had dropped so low that the crimson syrup did not so much flow into the collecting tube, as it did squirt in discreet pulses, like milk from a hand-squeezed udder. Tomorrow, David, having received the results, would post on his blog, "Good news! James's urine tested negative for amphetamines, barbiturates, benzodiazepine, marijuana, cocaine, opiates, and phencyclidine. He did, however, test positive for *crazy sonofabitch.*"

I went into Izzy's house and laid on a table so that Derek, a local chiropractor, could treat my war-torn body. 1, 2, 3, and I was sound asleep on his treatment table. He worked on me, as I slept deeply, for the next hour before it was time to get on my bike.

While I rode my bike through Iredell County, my kids played on a swing set on Izzy's property, watched over by Izzy's friend Meghan. As the children swooped back and forth in wider and wider arcs, seemingly fearless, Meghan moved by their banter, which seemed to her to have a second layer of meaning beneath the superficial.

How high can you go?
As high as that bush!
As high as that tree!
As high as the sky!

Hearing this story later brought a smile to my face. In some ways, I felt, I wasn't living up to my usual standards as a father on this journey. I had so little time and

energy for the kids while I was out here on the Fifty. My hope was that this temporary freeze in our time together was overridden by the example I was setting. The
swing-set incident suggested it just might be. Perhaps it was in part by watching me
that Quinn and the girls had come to believe the sky was the limit—literally.

My hamstring tendon gave me trouble from the very first pedal stroke and got
worse and worse as I continued riding with about eighty supporters. Less than twenty miles in, I peeled away from the group. Only my guide, Blake, followed me.

"I'm in pain," I told him.

Blake called Derek, the chiropractor who had treated me at Izzy's house, and
asked him to meet us ASAP at Jetton Park, where we were staging. Derek was waiting for us when we got there.

I sat down on the ground and Derek knelt to have a look. He squeezed the calf
muscle and asked if it hurt. I shook my head no. He moved his hands up a few inches
and squeezed again. This time he didn't have to ask. I groaned and reached out reflexively to pry Derek's talons off me, but he let go first.

"How about when I do this?" he asked, grasping my shank and bending my
knee. I squeezed my eyes shut and inhaled sharply through clenched teeth.

"Oh, my gosh!" said Derek.

These words are ones you never want to hear a medical professional utter while
examining your body. I had heard them twice so far in the Fifty—first from Karen in
Mississippi, when she saw my toe blister, and now from Derek, who had never seen
so light a touch cause so intense a reaction.

"Do you think this could have anything to do with a blood clot?" I asked, almost whispering. Derek paused—too long, I felt—before answering.

"No, I don't," he said.

"So what's the worst thing that could happen?" I asked.

"You could tear that tendon off the bone, and you'd be completely unable to use
your leg."

I sagged with relief. *Tear the tendon off the bone?* I thought. *That's it?* A severed
tendon could heal, and in the meantime, I could pedal with one leg if I had to. But a
blood clot was death. *Game on!*

Dispensing with the advice he surely would have given anyone else in my condition—"Don't you *dare* get back on that bike!"—Derek wrapped the knee, and I
resumed my ride. It took me about three seconds to realize I could not pedal comfortably with my knee wrapped. As soon as I was out of sight, I stopped, undid Der-

7 ANOTHER DAY, ANOTHER DIAGNOSIS

ek's careful work, and tossed the bandage in a dumpster.

I got through the last ninety miles in the only way possible—by not thinking about them. My singular goal was to survive one more minute. That much I knew I could do. When the minute was up, I set the same goal for the next minute. After 327 minutes, I was done.

The ride ended at Podium Multisport, a hub of the Charlotte area's triathlon community. Aaron led me to a changing room at the back of the store and handed me my running gear. I asked him to fetch my knee brace, which I'd worn only once before, in Flagstaff, with disastrous results. I was desperate.

"How is it?" Aaron asked, wincing empathetically.

"It hurts," I said.

"What's it going to be like to run on it?" he asked.

"Slow," I said.

A slow marathon would mean a late finish, and a late finish would mean the motor home—and my family—would have to leave ahead of me yet again, and I would have to sleep on the floor of the van. Again.

"I'd really like Sunny to stay behind with me," I told Aaron. "I know she won't want to, but do you think you can talk her into it?"

Up to this point in the campaign, Sunny had refused to let the kids travel alone in the motor home with Casey driving. He'd had a few close calls, and with a mother's logic, she was convinced that her absence from the motor home would make an accident inevitable. She had also driven many nights, offering Casey relief so that he could catch a short nap before starting his hectic day. Even at that, right now I needed the sort of comfort that only she could give me.

Dressed to run, I moved to the front of the store and laid face up on a waiting massage table to get a little bodywork from someone Izzy had found for me. Sunny and the kids, who had just arrived from Izzy's, filtered in and surrounded me, having just learned of my latest crisis. Lucy, brow furrowed, placed a soothing hand on my forehead.

The marathon took place in Jetton Park, where my supporters and I traced 1.5-mile loops around Lake Norman, pausing at the end of each to take refreshments from Izzy. A guy named Chris had driven from Virginia to attempt his very first marathon at my side. He was full of questions.

"Why are you wearing two watches?" he asked early on.

"In case something happens to one of them," I said. "I need proof of every step I take, or people will say I didn't really do it."

The various Internet forums focused on the Fifty had been overrun by anti–Iron Cowboy vitriol since Elliptigate, and although I tried to tune it out, some of the venoms filtered back to me, and the haters were always lurking in the back of my mind.

Kelly, a professional triathlete, somehow got me onto the topic of life after the Fifty, which I typically tried to avoid. I told her I wanted to travel to schools all across America and speak about childhood obesity. Kelly suggested I take a long break before I tackled any other major undertakings and worried aloud that I would experience "post-Ironman blues"—a well-documented phenomenon—"times fifty."

"If I were you, I would consider getting some counseling," she said.

"That's a good idea," I said.

In truth, Kelly's advice irritated me. I thought, *How could a person strong enough to survive the Fifty possibly struggle afterward?* I was that naive.

With four miles to go, Kelly and I bumped elbows and my primary watch stopped.

"See what I mean?" I said to Chris.

It was past one o'clock in the morning when I returned to Izzy's house to shower before hitting the road. Aaron had succeeded in talking Sunny into staying back with me, and she was still awake. I could tell right away from her pursed lips and clipped speech that something was eating at her. I tried to play dumb, but that never works.

"How was your day?" I asked searchingly.

"We had a fun day!" she said.

"We went to a petting zoo, but this was no ordinary petting zoo; there were water buffalo, an ostrich, and other exotic animals. We rode in a large wagon, they passed out buckets of food, and we were able to feed the animals. The kids absolutely LOVED it!"

I could tell that Sunny was focusing on the positive part of the day; after all, she was always grateful when activities were provided for her to do with the kids, with little or no effort.

She explained that after the petting zoo, they returned to Izzy's place, when she started to answer emails and fell asleep on a sofa, completely worn out. Sunny had been focused and diligent this whole journey, and I can only imagine how exhausted she was every day.

"When I woke up, I could smell dinner cooking. I walked up the stairs and could hear the beef sizzling on the skillet."

Izzy's wife, Stephanie, was preparing tacos, a Lawrence family favorite. When Stephanie had asked for requests earlier that day, it was a simple; a home-cooked meal was all that the family wanted. Between the sizzling beef, the TV, and children's voices (Izzy and Stephanie had two of their own), Sunny had a realization.

"Today is the first day that I miss home."

She finally opened up about her struggles that day, and thus far on the Fifty, struggles that she had tried to avoid mentioning to me, not wanting to increase my burdens. I listened, we acknowledged and appreciated our 15 minutes alone (which never happened on the Fifty), and then we headed out to the car.

8

ASSAULT ON IMPOSSIBLE

2013–2015
UTAH

In the spring of 2013, about six months after I set my second world record, my friend Steve, a Lindon City police officer, was looking for someone to help care for his mother, being that she lived alone. Joyce, who was afflicted with Alzheimer's disease, needed some assisted care, and the family wanted someone to move in with her. The timing was perfect for us, as was this new job, being that things had escalated with our landlords, and bad situations had gotten worse. We had reached our wits end after our landlords had been persistent in their efforts to drive us out by putting up fences to block us from our yard, constantly harassing us with potential contract breeches, and only heating part of the house, which forced our kids to sleep next to the fireplace to stay warm at night. We now had an opportunity to leave this experience behind, and bless Joyce's life. We were thrilled and couldn't wait for moving day.

A few months after we moved in with Joyce, a package arrived with my name on it. Its dimensions hinted at something like a baseball bat, but it was very light. Opening it, I found a rolled-up three-foot-by-four-foot map of the United States that I'd ordered online. I took it straight down to the basement, where Sunny and I shared a tiny room that served as bedroom and office. At the foot of the staircase was an even smaller space that the family used as a central gathering point. I tacked the map to a wall there.

After initial disbelief and convincing me to postpone it from 2014 to 2015, Sunny had agreed to support me in pursuing my vision of completing fifty iron-distance triathlons, in fifty states, in fifty days, but only on the condition that I do all the planning myself. She was finishing up her bachelor's degree in psychology at Utah Valley University, caring for Joyce, volunteering with church youth groups, and taking care of our family.

The map's purpose was not so much to aid in this planning as to make the project concrete and real for the kids. Over the ensuing months, we would have many a conversation about what each state was like (or at least what it was known for) and what they wished to do there while Daddy was busy swimming, cycling, and running. Sunny and I wanted each child to feel fully involved at every step. For this same reason, I had decided to undertake the mission in the summer of 2015, when school was out for summer break.

Around the time the map went up, I invited my friend and on-and-off coach David out for breakfast at Kneaders Bakery. We settled into a booth where David ordered French toast, and I went for the usual, omelet with broccoli, and a side of fruit. While we ate, I laid out my latest scheme, speaking low and fast, as though fearful of being either overheard or timed out. David listened with a faint smile frozen on his face, regarding me like a freshly paroled bank robber detailing his next big heist.

"Well, what do you think?" I concluded.

"I think it's absolutely amazing," David said. "You've set an incredible goal. I really admire your vision."

"But you don't think I can do it."

"I don't think *anyone* can do fifty Ironmans, in fifty states, in fifty days," David said. "Don't take it personally."

I reminded David I had proven him wrong twice already, with each of my world records.

"I know it's a huge leap," I said, "but I honestly think it's possible. Not without you, though. I don't need you to believe in me. I just need you to coach me."

David agreed to coach me. Then he got right down to it, hitting me with a series of good questions, most of them concerning the logistical side of the venture. He asked how I would handle Alaska and Hawaii, given their remoteness. I told him I would attempt them first, so if something went wrong, I could easily reset and start over. He asked what criteria I would use to select my swim, bike, and run courses. I told him that I would look on Google Earth, and then recruit one or more ambassadors in each state to make sure the routes I picked were well suited for my specific circumstances.

"You're really going to do this?" he asked as we left the restaurant.

"Yes, *we* really are," I said.

My breakfast with David took place only days after I had decided to pull out of Ironman Cozumel. I had a nagging muscle strain in my lower abdomen that made running impossible and cycling unpleasant. I decided to only complete the Cozumel swim, since I had paid the race entry fee, and called it a day before the bike and run. Two months earlier, the same injury had forced me to walk the entire marathon at Ironman Lake Tahoe. David knew all about these recent struggles, so when he told me he didn't think I could complete fifty iron-distance triathlons in as many days, he was fully aware that he was talking to a man who was currently incapable of finishing *one* iron-distance triathlon.

I had cause for hope, though. At the beginning of the year, I had begun to work with a new chiropractor, Dallas. The man possessed an incredible knowledge of kinesiology, sports injuries, and techniques for treating and preventing them. My appointments with him not only eased my aches and pains, but they also taught me about my body and how to challenge its limits without exceeding them. After several months in his care, I had not yet turned the corner with my abdominal injury, but I felt confident that when I did, I would be much less likely to suffer future break-downs.

At the height of my training for the Fifty, Dallas, and my longtime friend and massage therapist, Natalie, would have their hands on me at least twice, and more often three times, a week. I considered these sessions to be just as important as my swims, bike rides, and runs. In fact, I might have given up swimming before I gave up Dallas and Natalie.

What I was most concerned about was how I would keep my body together during the Fifty. It was clear to me that if I had little chance of starting it without these two wizards, I had zero chance of finishing it on my own. I decided to pitch each of them on coming along with me, but for both family and work reasons neither could commit to the full tour. In the end, Natalie agreed to drop in on me twice (Days 3 through 6 and Days 47 through 50) and I convinced Dallas to fly out and support me on five of the seven weekends while I was on the road. I could only hope this would suffice.

In January 2014, my coach had a training plan for me. David likes to do things by the book, but there was no book for what I was attempting, so he had to wing it. With sixteen months to fill before my quest began, he suggested we divide the preparatory process into two phases. In the first phase, I would be using traditional methods, pursue a goal that's on every serious triathlete's bucket list: competing in the Ironman World Championship in Kona, Hawaii. Then I would transition to specific training for the Fifty.

In this second phase, I would need to simulate the challenges I would face in the Fifty by routinely training for several hours on successive days. David and I both knew that trying to simulate the Fifty too closely was risky, and would potentially destroy me. By David's reckoning, the sweet spot between under preparation and self-destruction was five- to seven-day cycles in which I would work out all day for three or four days, and then recuperate for two or three days. Almost everything I did would be executed at a crawling pace; after all, I wasn't going for a speed record.

"It's going to be really, really boring," David said.

The fact that David thought it unwise for me to exercise for more than ten hours in a day for more than four straight days gave me pause. My goal was to exercise for *fourteen* hours a day for *fifty* days. Contemplating the vast mathematical gulf that existed between my preparation and the thing I was preparing for caused me to experience the first "Oh crap," moment I'd had since dreaming up the Fifty, and it would definitely not be the last.

Including strength workouts (which would entail a mix of the basic functional stuff that David liked, and the CrossFit-type stuff that I loved and David pooh-poohed), I would be training for thirty-two hours a week in my heaviest weeks. These hours would have to fit around my family responsibilities that always came first, not to mention the daunting work of planning the logistics of the Fifty and running its business side.

Phase One ended with an ill-timed blow to my confidence. Despite solid preparation, I raced poorly in Kona, getting blown all over the bike course by the island's infamous *Mumuku* winds and spending more time throwing up than running during the marathon. I finished 1,536th out of 2,118 starters.

On to Phase Two. It took a little time, but eventually, I settled into a routine that balanced everything optimally, if not perfectly. Twice a week I took Daisy and Lily with me to five thirty a.m. group swim workouts. On the other weekdays, I let myself sleep a little longer (but not much) and squeezed in a short workout in the Shred Shed—a detached garage on Joyce's property that Sunny and I had cleaned out and converted into a private indoor cycling studio—before the kids woke. At eight thirty, I threw together a breakfast of scrambled eggs and hash browns for everyone, and then I drove the girls to school. Some days Sunny took Quinn to class with her, where he sat through her classes with extraordinary patience. Other days we got our friend Carlee to look after him, but more often than not, though, I kept him with me.

While the girls were at school, I packed in as much training and computer time as I could. Quinn's contended nature made this easier than it would have been with most five-year-olds. He could entertain himself with toys and his imagination for hours while I pedaled away in the Shred Shed. He loved swinging on the rings and bars, doing flips on the mats, or just bringing toys out to play in the shed. He would have play dates with other kids a few days a week as well, to break up the monotony. Every once in a while, he would come to my desk with a box of LEGO or his Tinkertoys and ask me to play with him. When his timing was poor—when Daddy was freaked out because Life Time Fitness had rejected a sponsorship proposal or because he couldn't find an ambassador for California (the center of the freaking triathlon universe!)—I might groan inwardly, but I never groaned outwardly. I always dropped what I was doing to give Quinn the quality time he deserved, even just 10-15 minutes made the difference. I found that I too, needed this time with him. There was a sign on a wall in our cramped basement kitchen that I saw several times every day: NO SUCCESS CAN COMPENSATE FOR FAILURE IN THE HOME.

When I needed to get in an extensive block of training, I got out of Dodge. My first big training camp took place at the end of February 2015, exactly one hundred days before the start of the Fifty. On the first day, I woke up early and swam 3,500 yards—a bit less than the Ironman distance—at Sand Hollow Aquatic Center. After a short break, I rode my bike for five hours and then ran for ninety minutes on the Ironman 70.3 St. George racecourse. The next day, I swam the same distance and rode another five hours, but covered nine fewer miles than I had in the same amount of time the day before. I was completely fried. But I wasn't done—I had a two-hour run ahead of me.

My ride ended at a house belonging to a friend's parents, where I was staying. I stumbled inside, peeled off my jersey, dropped the straps of my bib shorts (my hosts were out), and heated up a Cup Noodles in the microwave. When the soup was hot, I took it into the TV room and sat down on a reclining chair upholstered in a nice, burgundy-colored leather. I slurped up the soup and then decided to rest my eyes for a minute.

I was woken two hours later by the laughing entrance of several people who had come to join me for the second half of my training camp: Sunny, Carlee, Natalie, a couple of athletes I coached, and Aaron, a newly recruited wingman for the Fifty. I leaped up from my seat in embarrassment. When the others saw the state I was in, they fell silent. I saw their eyes wander over to the expensive piece of furniture I had just napped on, sweaty and shirtless. I turned around and discovered it was covered in a film of salt in the shape of my body.

"Dang, I hope that comes out," I said.

I rallied as best I could and ran ten miles. The next day, I broke from my plan and trained with the girls instead of the guys. I could barely keep up with Sunny and her friends. My confidence was now thoroughly shattered. David was right. What I was preparing to do truly was impossible. I felt a powerful temptation to back out, but it was too late. My pride was now on the line.

I was still reeling from my disastrous training camp when I flew to Los Angeles a week later to sit down for an interview about the Fifty with Rich Roll, a famous ultra-endurance athlete and the host of a popular fitness and nutrition podcast.

"You're ninety days out," Rich said midway through our conversation. "How are you feeling?"

"I'm terrified," I said.

The interview was posted on Rich's website under the title *Assault on Impossible*, generating a buzz in the endurance community and deepening my terror. It's one thing to fail; it's quite another to fail famously.

It fell largely on David's shoulders to make me less terrified. A good coach is as much a therapist as he is a workout planner. David wasn't just a good coach, but a great one. When I told him about the recliner episode, he expressed neither surprise nor concern, a reaction that immediately lowered my anxiety level.

"Two things," he said. "First, you went into the camp already tired. You need to back off before the next one."

"And the second thing?" I asked.

"You're still going too fast," David said. "You need to go slower—I mean painfully slow. If you do that, you'll find the workouts a lot more manageable."

I knew David was right, but what he was asking me to do defied every racer's instincts. The previous year, when I had been focused on preparing for the Ironman World Championship, my training had been all about getting faster. Now I had to replace my racer's mindset with its opposite—to become the master of the eleven-minute mile, as it were.

The longer I kept holding myself back in my subsequent training, though, the easier it became psychologically to continue doing so. As David had predicted, I felt less overwhelmed by the long hours. In the middle of March, now less than twelve weeks before the start of the Fifty, I returned to St. George for a second big training camp. I completed twenty-six total hours of exercise in three days and handled it well. The difference between these figures and those I would accumulate in the Fifty still turned my stomach inside out, but both my fitness and my confidence were moving in the right direction.

On May 25, 2015, the day before I flew to Hawaii with my family to begin the Fifty, I sat down with David for another breakfast at Kneaders.

"Do you still say it's impossible?" I asked.

"I'm really impressed by what you were able to do in your training," he said. "You've come a long way—further than I expected."

"But you still don't think I can do it."

"I give you a 20 percent chance. Up from zero."

"I'm going to enjoy proving you wrong again," I said.

"Nothing would make me happier," David said.

We shook hands and parted.

The next morning, my family and I loaded our luggage and ourselves into a fifteen-passenger van that my biggest sponsor, Young Living, had purchased for the Fifty. We had vacated Joyce's house six weeks before and were now staying with our friend Liz, all our worldly possessions jammed inside her extra garage. My buddy Ed met us there to drive us to the airport. Afterward, he would return the van to Liz's house, where my crew would collect it ten days later and deliver it to our Day 3 meeting point in Seattle.

As we headed north on I-15 through light rain, I brooded on several worries, my fitness being least among them. A number of other elements of the campaign had failed to come together as I'd hoped and were causing me no small amount of eleventh-hour heartburn.

Worry number one was the motor home situation. Months before, the Fifty's project manager, Jordan, a young entrepreneur and a former client of mine, had landed a deal with Fleetwood RV to supply a motor home to serve as the campaign's flagship in the Lower Forty-Eight. The company's CEO had agreed to hand over a thirty-foot Class C Storm after a NASCAR event in Utah in April. This would leave me with plenty of time to have the vehicle wrapped in Iron Cowboy branding and sponsor logos. But then the CEO resigned suddenly to care for his ailing wife, and the new management refused to honor our arrangement.

Just ten days before we were to fly out to Hawaii, Jordan tracked down the former CEO through Twitter and talked him into pleading our case with his late employer. His efforts succeeded, more or less, but under the new arrangement, we were required to fetch the motor home from Fleetwood's headquarters in Indiana.

Aaron volunteered for the mission. Like Jordan, Aaron had first come to me as a client. Impressed by his cycling prowess, I later recruited him to join Sunny, wingman Casey, and me on a relay team I put together for the Saints to Sinners Bike Relay (which goes from Salt Lake City to Las Vegas—get it?). Sunny pegged Casey as the perfect wingman candidate when, after we had won the event, he climbed onto the roof of our van wearing pink booty shorts and hollered into a megaphone. Aaron had a similar kind of playful energy, and the two of them, though they had just met, keyed off each other like a veteran comedy duo. I wanted both of them, and I got them. Aaron quit a job with JetBlue for the gig, and Casey, a teacher with summers off, got an extended hall pass from his wife, Ryanne, who would stay home to look after their three young children.

On May 27—the next day—Aaron and his father would board a flight to Indianapolis and then drive the RV nonstop back to Utah, where I'd found a guy who was willing (for the right price) to wrap it in half the usual time. When the job was completed, the two wingmen would take the motor home to Liz's house and load it up with all my gear and supplies for the Fifty. If absolutely nothing went wrong, they would leave for our rendezvous point in Washington on June 6, the same day I was to start the Fifty in Hawaii.

Weighing almost as heavily on me was the charity situation. I had decided very early in the process of planning the Fifty that I wanted to attach it to a cause that meant something to me personally. While I had felt good about raising money for water projects in Kenya, I had never been to the country, and I did not know any Kenyan people. Through my kids, I came face-to-face almost every day with an immense problem that touched me directly: childhood obesity.

🎱 ASSAULT ON IMPOSSIBLE

An alarmingly large number of Lucy, Lily, Daisy, Dolly, and Quinn's playmates and classmates were overweight. The cause was no great mystery to me. Almost every overweight kid I encountered had parents who ate poorly and didn't move enough. Eating better and moving more are difficult changes to make, and they seem downright impossible to many people. In doing the humanly impossible in the Fifty, and in linking the Fifty to the cause of childhood obesity, I wanted to make such changes seem even more possible to those who struggled with them.

I began to look into charities that addressed childhood obesity. This search led me to Jamie Oliver, a British celebrity chef, and restaurateur who had thrown himself into the cause that was now my cause. I became an instant fan when I found and watched a prize winning TED Talk Jamie had given in 2010. I loved his in-your-face style, which I intended to draw inspiration from in the speech I gave each day before the Iron Cowboy 5K.

Despite my prior work for In Our Own Quiet Way, I still knew next to nothing about nonprofit fund-raising, and my naiveté was costing me. After a phone conversation with the Jamie Oliver Food Foundation, we knew that they were on board. When they failed to follow through on what was originally committed, I decided to press ahead and raise money for them anyway, both by taking donations on my website and passing along any donations that came from the Iron Cowboy 5K registrations. What I had hoped for was that the success of my rogue fund-raising efforts would please the Jamie Oliver Food Foundation, and motivate them to provide the link that they had agreed to create for my website. They would continue to ignore us in our attempts to contact them during the Fifty.

Then there was the documentary film situation. Creating a commercial-quality video record of the Fifty was important for a couple of reasons. It would expand the campaign's reach in space and time and offer further exposure to my sponsors. I had found the perfect crew for the job, but they weren't cheap. Months of solicitations had failed to produce an investor, and I was almost out of time. If I couldn't get the film made, not only would I not have the movie, but I might also lose other sponsors.

Just two weeks before, I reached out to Vaughn Cook, the CEO of ZYTO, a newer sponsor, and asked him if he knew anyone who might be willing to finance the documentary. Vaughn told me he'd see what he could do. Since then, I had still heard nothing from Vaughn. Minutes before we reached the airport, my phone rang. It was Vaughn.

"I think I have a solution for you," he said. "I'm going to pay for the documentary myself. Who should I make the check out to?"

I turned to Sunny and mouthed a single word: "Yes!" In an instant, my list of worries had shrunk by one item. Suddenly I felt assured that the other problems hanging over me would work themselves out as well. The RV would be wrapped and ready for me in Seattle and The Jamie Oliver Food Foundation would come around before the Fifty officially began.

My thoughts immediately shifted to the ten-day family vacation on the island of Kauai that I had very wisely planned as a calm before the storm of my quest.

Ed dropped us off at Terminal 2. We checked in (always an adventure with five young children) and made our way to the gate. On the way, we bumped into none other than Rich Roll, Mr. Assault on Impossible himself, who was heading back home to Los Angeles after an event in our area.

"How are you feeling now?" he asked, referring to my previous answer to the same question.

"Two hundred percent!" I said.

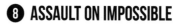 8 ASSAULT ON IMPOSSIBLE

HOW ARE YOU EVEN ALIVE?

DAYS 25–26
VIRGINIA, WEST VIRGINIA

"You're almost halfway. How has it been so far?"

The question came from Makenzie, a reporter for WTKR television who'd way-laid me the moment I dragged myself out of the van at Jamestown Beach Event Park in Williamsburg, Virginia, in desperate need of the nearest bathroom.

"It's as hard as I thought it was going to be," I answered, my attention equally divided between my interviewer and my sphincter. "On the other hand, I'm super stoked to be feeling the way I do halfway through. We've made it through what I think are the hardest stretches with the biggest obstacles and my body's adjusting."

Had Mackenzie known the full extent of the ailments that underlay this self-as-sessment- chronic fatigue, extreme sleep deprivation, sore tongue, thrush, shredded right shoulder, bloated gut, abdominal strain, bruised right hip, saddle sores, bloody stools, tender and cramp-prone inner thigh muscles, severe hamstring tendonitis, and gruesome toe blisters-she would have thought that I was insane. But what I meant by "adjusting" was that most of these ailments were actually getting better, not worse, and that's all that mattered to me. I never expected to get through the Fifty unscarred.

Eleven cyclists set out from the park with me after my swim in the James River. Within an hour, eight of them had left me in their dust.

"I've got this thing on the back of my knee," I'd told them before we started, "so I might be a little slower than normal."

Informing them of this pain was my way of encouraging patience, but it was interpreted, apparently, as permission to go on ahead and let me fend for myself. My remaining three supporters, lacking the fitness to ride the full distance, turned around at fifteen miles, leaving me alone with Walt, a young bike mechanic tailing me in a Mercedes-Benz cargo van he'd rigged up as a mobile bicycle repair shop. That's when the tunnel vision started. Suddenly it felt as though I'd overdosed on a powerful sleep medication that was seeping into my brain and dragging my consciousness under with implacable chemical force. Keeping my eyelids open was akin to arm-wrestling a clone, requiring unflagging effort and absolute concentration to achieve no better result than an eternal stalemate. I nodded off a few times despite these mental exertions and woke up once to find myself veering into the busy northbound traffic lane on Route 5.

My entire body clenched in raw terror. I felt absurdly powerless to act for my own self-preservation. All I had to do was stay awake, but I couldn't! At twenty-five miles, my rattled nerves were shot. Heart thudding, I pulled onto the shoulder and waved Walt forward.

He slid open the van's side door and helped me climb in. Having explained my situation, I sat on the floor, folded my arms over my knees, and let my head drop. Suddenly more hungry than sleepy, I emptied my jersey pockets of all the food I'd stuffed in them and ate it, chasing the meal with a Chocolate Protein Monster Energy Drink.

I waited—and prayed—for the caffeine and calories to kick in. Five minutes passed. Nothing. Ten minutes. Nada. Despair settled over me like a chill. At no point in the campaign had I felt more alone or trapped than I did now. None of my people knew where I was or what was happening to me and the clock was ticking. I had to get back out on the road soon, but I was afraid to try, certain I would nod off one time too many and topple into the path of an oncoming Cadillac Escalade. I went back and forth in my mind, deciding first to wait, then to go for it, then to wait. A sudden impulse broke the cycle.

"Come here," I said to Walt. "Let's take a picture."

I pointed to the spot where I wanted him to crouch, angled my phone just so, and captured the image.

"You've got to take the bad with the good," I said. "I want this picture to help me remember what the bad felt like."

I got out of the van and got back on my bike—still tired, still scared, but now accepting my predicament that rest and nutrition had failed to fix it. Nothing physical could fix it. The one thing I could control was my attitude, so I decided the predicament was a test rather than a setback. Unable to change my situation, I changed its meaning instead, embracing the idea that today it was not meant for me to conquer the source of my fear but to face my fear—to keep believing and take the next step despite it.

When I returned to the staging area several hours later, I was in a funny mood—the sort of reflective, appreciative mood that sometimes follows a scare. I sat outside the motor home watching Aaron hustle to get my running gear together, his expression earnest, his movements hurried but careful, like those of a proud sous chef at a bustling restaurant. This man did not want to fail me.

"You know I love you, right?" I said.

Aaron froze like a scolded child.

"I love you too, man," he said cautiously.

"No, I'm serious," I said. "I appreciate everything you're doing."

"Thanks," Aaron said. "I'm just happy to be out here."

My peculiar mental state followed me to Jamestown High School, where we staged for the marathon. Night fell as I ran the first of several post-5K loops around the Greensprings Greenway Interpretive Trail with six or seven supporters. Meanwhile, back at the high school parking lot, a dance party broke out. Someone cranked the volume on a car stereo, others produced flashlights, a bike light (set in strobe mode, naturally), and a glow stick or two. When I came upon the scene, Casey, Aaron, and even Quinn—none of whom needs any excuse to shake a tail feather—were grooving alongside several locals to David Guetta's "Hey Mama."

A giddy impulse rose up in me. I bounded into the center of the circle and began to do something that felt (and probably looked) like a cross between a rain dance and the funky chicken. The others laughed and cheered. Casey, flabbergasted, just stared, briefly neglecting his own dancing. This was the first truly silly thing he'd seen me do in twenty-five days—the first time I had voluntarily *wasted energy*. Like my earlier decision to get back on my bike and ride through crushing tiredness and paralyzing fear, it just felt right. Instinct assured me I wasn't really wasting energy; I was *giving* energy to my family, my crew, and my supporters—and getting it right back.

During the next lap around the trail, a dramatic lightning storm came out of nowhere to unleash chaos all around us, and I now had another tough decision to make. After Elliptigate, I had vowed to do no more indoor cycling or running, but if

I continued to run outdoors now, others would insist on staying with me. If one of those others got him- or herself electrocuted, it would be my fault, so I reluctantly decided to finish the marathon under a roof.

Earlier in the evening, a young man named David had leaped out of a slow-moving car to join our group. He'd cut an impressive figure as he dashed toward us with bouncing dreadlocks and a ropy physique that combined a powerlifter's muscularity and an ultrarunner's leanness. I soon learned that David was, in fact, a powerlifter and an ultrarunner and that he worked at a local physical therapy facility. I now asked him, between claps of thunder, if he had any treadmills there.

"I've got three," he said. "And one of them has your name on it."

We hustled through pelting rain to the staging area, where I said good night and goodbye to Sunny and the kids, who would soon roll out toward West Virginia. David took the wheel of the same car he'd leaped out of an hour before and led the way to the Williamsburg Neck and Back Center. I settled into the front passenger seat of a Honda Element driven by my Virginia ambassador, Valerie. She had been with me most of the day, plying me with pancakes and eggs after I swam, shaking rainbow-colored cowbells as I passed her at various points of my bike ride, and now staying up late to play "follow that car."

Full-figured and coffee-complected, Valerie did not resemble the archetypal triathlete, and yet she had completed more than one Ironman. She had greeted me with an enigmatic smile this morning as I sat in the van eating oatmeal while Sunny rubbed my feet—a smile that seemed to express a mixture of warmth and self-consciousness. Here, in the privacy of her vehicle, Valerie opened up to me about her struggle to overcome lifelong insecurities through triathlon.

"I've always been heavy," she said, "even though I've always done sports."

Valerie graduated from high school as a top performer on the swim team and weighing 250 pounds. A lengthy period of relative inactivity and unhappiness followed, but then she discovered triathlon and was reborn.

"It's not about weight management for me," she said. "It's not about getting faster. I do it for how it makes me feel, and the sense of community, and the travel, and the opportunity to just get outside and enjoy nature."

Although Valerie couldn't help but wish all her training had made her skinny, it hadn't. This disappointment was more than made up for, however, by everything else the sport had given her. And she was wise enough to recognize that looking different from other triathletes allowed her to give back to the sport in a way she could not have done if she blended in with everyone else.

"I want people to see a big, brown girl on the starting line," she told me.

"I think you're beautiful," I said.

We arrived at David's facility and went in. I hopped aboard the middle treadmill, a woman named Monica chose the machine to my left, and David claimed the one in the corner. A couple of others who'd tagged along, Libida and Bernie, waited for their turns. The ZYTO girls, Sariah and Hannah, arrived a short time later with pillows clasped to their chests and, with unnecessary apologies, asked for a place to lie down. David showed them to a backroom containing treatment beds.

Valerie had brought along a speaker system. David plugged in his phone and asked what I wanted to hear.

"Got any 50 Cent?" I asked.

I wasn't trying to score cool points. Rap had been my go-to "finishing music" throughout the campaign. Valerie put it on, but kept the volume at a moderate level that allowed the ZYTO girls to sleep and the rest of us to converse. I continued to feel vaguely intoxicated, and the buzz made me unusually talkative. I recounted the story of my Ferris wheel adventure, described the night I was rolled out of the E Center in a wheelchair, and shared some of the challenges and setbacks I had experienced both before and during the Fifty.

"One thing I've learned," I said as I neared the end of my night's labors, "is that there's always a way to get to the other side of the mountain. Sometimes you have to go up and over, and other times you have to take the long way around. Once in a while, you have to tunnel right through the sucker, but there's always a way."

Nobody said anything for a moment or two, then David spoke. "You're kind of a spiritual dude, aren't you?" he said.

I laughed, a little embarrassed, but then I thought about David's remark. Is it a spiritual thing to trust that life's challenges will always work themselves out if you just believe and never quit? Maybe so.

Marathon completed, David guided me to the shower room. The water was hot, and the pressure was excellent. I closed my eyes and let the hot spray massage my skin. Only then did I realize I was exactly halfway through my mission.

IRON COWBOY

Jamie greeted me with a painfully firm handshake, the kind that seems intended to assert dominance.

"How's the water?" I asked my West Virginia ambassador.

"It's warm," he said.

I didn't believe him. The chill of an unseasonably cool night still lingered in the air at Cheat Lake in east Morgantown more than an hour after sunrise. I sensed that Jamie had no actual knowledge that the water was warm—that he would answer any question I asked with the words he thought I wanted to hear.

We had almost canceled our visit to Morgantown late yesterday in favor of throwing together an improvised triathlon in the southern part of the state, which was a lot closer not only to the previous day's triathlon venue in Williamsburg, but also to Cambridge, Maryland, where we were scheduled to be tomorrow. Jamie had convinced us to stick with plan A, promising tons of local support and a big media turnout, neither of which was evident yet.

Despite my skepticism, I put on my sleeveless wetsuit. Bill and Jason, who had stepped forward to offer their services as swim guides, led me to the beach. I took one step into the lake and froze.

"You call this warm?" I asked.

Bill and Jason shrugged. I told them I'd be right back and stormed away to the RV to pull on my full wetsuit.

A few people had come out to swim with me or just to watch. Returning to the water's edge, I overheard a couple of women wearing wetsuits talking nervously about the prospect of covering 2.4 miles in open water, something neither of them had done before.

"Just get in and give it a shot," I said. "What's the worst that could happen?"

"We could drown," they said.

Well, sure, but they gave it a shot anyway, and although one of the two turned around early (and wisely, no doubt), the other hung on the whole way. The thousand-watt smile that lit up her face when she came out of the water was my vindication for challenging her, and her reward for accepting the challenge.

My swimming experience was not without its challenges. Casey had been unable to find the anti-chafe cream I used whenever I wore a wetsuit. He ransacked the motor home and the van and the family Mazda we'd been towing behind it in a rising panic, but came up empty. A local supporter then offered me a tub of Aquaphor as a substitute, and I slathered it on my friction areas. An oily residue still covered my

⑨ HOW ARE YOU EVEN ALIVE?

thumbs when I used them to rub spittle into my swim goggles to prevent fogging. I hadn't swum more than ten yards when I realized I couldn't see a dang thing. I heard Jason splashing to my left, and I felt Bill's slipstream in front of me, but I might as well have been looking at the world through wax paper.

I stopped swimming and trod water with my legs only (not easy) as I tried to wash the film of ointment off the lenses. Then I put the goggles on and started swimming again. Still wax paper. I stopped a second time.

"Here," Bill said. "Take these."

He handed me his goggles, and I gave him mine. Bill strapped the useless eyewear up around his forehead, intending to swim head-up. When I continued swimming, the borrowed goggles immediately filled with water and I was blind yet again. I have a very narrow face with deep eye sockets and a protruding brow, and only a few types of goggles fit me; these certainly didn't.

Treading water again, I noticed Casey and Aaron were watching us from a trestle bridge. I called out to them, and they ran off to fetch my reserve goggles. Bill swam back to shore to receive them while I made slow progress with unprotected eyes. Bill caught up to us with humbling ease, and for the remainder of the swim, my only worry was my plunging core body temperature. As my exposed skin went numb and my lips turned blue, I vowed I would never again take someone else's word about water temperature.

On land, the wingmen stripped off my wetsuit, bundled me in blankets, and tossed me in the back of the van with the heater on full blast. I was still shivering half an hour later when we arrived at the Seneca Center, a turn-of-the-century glass factory that had been converted into a retail space. Among its several tenants was a bike shop with a back patio that abutted the Caperton Trail, a rail trail that Jamie had chosen as my cycling venue.

Jamie now proudly introduced me to Nick, a reporter for Channel 12, the one and only representative of the press I would see today. Nick set up a camera, and I sat crossways on the top tube of my bike to answer his questions. My kids cruised around us on their bikes while Jordan, his wife Jessa's, and their two Pomeranians (yes, they'd brought their dogs on our expedition) scampered about with the same youthful energy.

"Which state has been your favorite so far?" Nick asked.

Not West Virginia, I thought. But I couldn't say that.

"Whatever place I'm in is my favorite," I said, "because it means I survived another day."

I was congratulating myself inwardly for this bit of diplomacy when the front wheel of my bike suddenly shifted, and I lost my balance. Nick leaped toward my flailing body with outstretched arms, but I recovered my equilibrium without aid and just in time to avoid landing painfully on top of my machine.

"Are you all right?" Nick asked.

"I'm sure I'll feel better after a six-hour bike ride," I quipped.

My six-hour bike ride began a few minutes later. Four locals started with me. We headed south on the rail trail, following the winding course of the Mononga-hela River. After six miles, we transitioned from pavement to crushed limestone. It might as well have been used kitty litter. Recent rainstorms had softened the surface and left the path dotted with invisible and treacherous compression dips—extra-soft patches where our front wheels sank in, threatening to send us somersaulting over the handlebars.

To make matters worse, the path was also strewn with debri—twigs, leaves, and branches that presumably had been brought down in the same recent storms. The five of us were forced to weave left and right and brake often to dodge the worst of the debris. We bumped wheels several times and were forced off the path altogether once or twice. While we escaped catastrophe, the effort required was physically and mentally draining. It was all too much like cycling through a minefield.

At the town of Fairmont, thirty miles from our starting point, we turned around. On the way back to the Seneca Center, I announced my intention to finish the ride by shuttling back and forth on the six-mile paved segment of the trail. Two of my companions agreed to stay with me. I can't say I would have done the same for them.

While I continued to work toward my 112-mile target, Sunny and the wingmen took care of the unglamorous behind-the-scenes duties that dominated their sched-ules. Like clothes washing. My daily exertions produced an astonishing amount of damp and pungent laundry, our children seemed to collect clothing stains intention-ally, and of course my wingmen were occupied with more important tasks, so Sunny did their laundry as well. On this particular day, virtually every item of apparel we'd brought on the trip was soiled and needed to be laundered. Jordan and Jessa had disappeared with the van, so Sunny had no other choice than to squeeze into the Mazda with all five kids, plus six heaping baskets of dirty garments, clown-car style. Casey slammed the driver door shut from the outside on a three count. Sunny drove

⑨ HOW ARE YOU EVEN ALIVE?

with a basket on her lap, eyes straining over piled-up sweaty socks. Naturally, the car was a stick shift.

Having seen my family safely off, Casey and Aaron tackled their chore for the day, getting an overdue oil change in the motor home. Jamie volunteered to guide the wingmen to the shop where he had his oil changes done. When they got there, however, the manager informed them that he "couldn't work on anything that big." As he spoke these words, two of his employees were working on a tractor-trailer cab right behind him. Aaron gestured over the manager's shoulder with his chin. The man turned around.

"That's different," he said.

Jamie, seeming to regard this rebuff as normal, said not to worry; he knew another place. But when Casey called that other place and explained what he needed, he was turned away again.

"Are you saying you *can't* do it or you *won't*?" Casey asked.

"Don't want to," drawled the voice on the other end.

Jamie said not to worry; he knew another place. This time they hit pay dirt, but they had to sit for a seeming eternity in a waiting room until the service was completed. Jamie filled the interval by telling the wingmen all about the time he ran across America. Aaron fell asleep somewhere around the Rockies.

When I had completed my bike ride, I clomped inside the Seneca Center and followed a labyrinthine hallway toward the bike shop in back. Coming around a corner, I nearly collided with my friend Haydn, who had just driven in from Pittsburgh, where he was working as a sports therapist for the Steelers football team. He'd already set up his treatment table right there in the hallway.

I felt a grin spread across my face. Haydn began to smile too, but the expression was abruptly interrupted by a look of alarm, which he tried to conceal by forcing a smile. I knew that expression; it was the expression people wear when they see someone they love who looks shockingly worse than he did the last time they saw him.

Haydn worked on me for the next twenty-five minutes, giving the greatest amount of attention to the painful lump on the back of my left knee. Meanwhile, Sunny, smelling like fabric softener, ran Dallas's cold laser over my hips and neck. When these treatments were finished, I went outside to the patio, where a throng of thirty or more Mountain Staters awaited the start of the Iron Cowboy 5K. I gave my usual speech, and then Jamie presented me with an autographed copy of *Freedom Run USA,* a self-published book chronicling his run across America. By the time I

107

completed my marathon with Jamie some six hours later, there was no longer any need for me to read it—he'd told me the whole story.

It was a cool, still night. A leafy western horizon had long since swallowed the sun, and the temperature had dropped below sixty. My family and the wingmen were on the road to Maryland. I woke up Hannah and Sariah, who were dozing in sleeping bags laid out next to the Subaru, and let them know I was done. While they packed up, I called Jordan and Jessa and asked them to fetch me. As we waited for them, I thanked Jamie and bid him farewell.

"I can't imagine what you're going through," he said.

"Sure you can," I said. "You ran across America."

"That was a joke compared to what you're doing," he said.

The van came and I loaded myself in. We drove five minutes to the Marriott where Haydn was staying, trailed by Jason, one of my swim guides from the morning, who had come back for the marathon and had volunteered to administer an IV, being vaguely qualified to do so.

We crowded into Haydn's suite. I took a long, hot shower and then lay down on the bed while my friend set up his table. Thirty seconds later, the table was ready, and I was fast asleep. Haydn woke me and told Jason to go ahead and stick me where I lay. His first attempt missed the mark and sent blood spewing all over the sheets.

"Good luck explaining that one!" I laughed.

Haydn never did get me onto his treatment table, instead working on me as best he could while I drifted in and out of sleep on his king-size bed. When it was time to go, my friend grabbed me by the shoulders and looked me dead in the eyes. "James, how are you doing, man?" he asked.

I understood what he really meant: "Level with me, James. How are you *really* doing?" But only later would Haydn confess how much more lay behind his words. Our earlier encounter inside the Seneca Center had left him shaken. I had seemed to him not only sick and weak but also *not quite there*. At that moment, he'd wanted to ask a different question than the one he'd just now uttered: "James, how are you even alive?" He'd resisted the impulse to speak these words, but he'd also made a mental note to watch me closely and to confront me if his second impression confirmed the first.

Haydn was fully prepared to demand that I abandon my mission if he didn't like what he saw from me here in his hotel room. Luckily, I was always at my best at the end of the day, so he elected not to intervene, instead, requesting only that I be

❾ HOW ARE YOU EVEN ALIVE?

straight with him.

"I'm good," I said, meeting his stare. "Don't worry about me. I've got this."

SO MUCH FOR THE PLAN

DAYS 1–5
HAWAII, ALASKA, WASHINGTON, OREGON, CALIFORNIA

A pulsing blue glow illuminated the darkness. I looked back and saw the flashing lights of a police car approaching in the distance at speed. My stomach turned a somersault. I told myself the cruiser was probably on its way to an accident and returned to minding the road ahead. But my gut knew otherwise.

The lights grew brighter, and then came a siren's wail. The police car drew up alongside our group of four, and a metallic voice crackled through a loudspeaker: "Pull over now!"

The cruiser shot ahead and veered onto the shoulder, forcing us to brake and dismount. The driver's side door flew open, and the officer stormed at us, mouth flapping. His words came in such a rapid torrent that most of them sailed right past me. I did catch something about complaints from motorists, which I thought this rather odd because it was three o'clock in the morning. I could not recall having seen more than two vehicles, besides the van my film crew was traveling in since we'd left the YMCA of Kauai an hour and fifteen minutes earlier.

"You have two choices," the cop concluded. "Get off the road now or spend the rest of the night in jail!"

I couldn't believe it. I was less than three hours into my fifty-day quest, and already I'd been thrown off script—perhaps irrecoverably. I pleaded with the cop, explaining what I was trying to accomplish and how important it was to me to be allowed to continue. We had tickets for a four thirty p.m. flight to Anchorage. If I failed to complete this first triathlon in time to claim my seat, the campaign would

111

be over almost before it had even started.

I might have saved my breath. The cop sneered at my appeal and repeated my options. He was beginning to work himself up into a fresh lather when Joe, one of two local guys in our group, cut him off.

"Hey, you can't talk to us like that!" he said. "We haven't done anything wrong. We're riding on the shoulder; we've got lights and reflectors—we're not breaking any laws. We have just as much right to be on this road as the drivers who complained about us."

Shut up, shut up, shut up, I thought as Joe spoke, but to my surprise, the cop did not tackle and cuff him but instead backed down. Grumbling one or two more half-hearted threats, he retreated to the cruiser to radio his dispatcher. While he was thus occupied, Joe pulled out his phone and mugged for a series of selfies with the police car in the background. Who was this guy?

When the cop came back to us from his vehicle, he behaved completely different from the way he had stormed at us initially. In a tone that was very nearly apologetic, he informed us that a cyclist had been killed on this very stretch of road recently and he was only concerned for our safety. After warning us not to let him catch my film crew taping on the move, he let us go. I nearly broke into tears with relief.

Several miles down the road, my front tire flatted. The others waited while I changed the tube, an operation that added ten minutes to the fifteen-minute time loss we'd already suffered.

"We're going to have to step it up a bit," I told my buddy Craig, who had come over from Oahu to support me.

We stepped it up. I knew David would have a fit when he saw the data from my power meter, which measured my pedaling effort in watts, but I felt I had no choice. The faster tempo proved too much for Joe, and he turned around. Half an hour later, my rear tire flatted. Having used the only spare tube I had, I borrowed Craig's. Back on the bike, I pedaled even harder. Rocky, the other local who'd been accompanying me, announced he'd had enough and also turned around, but not before he'd handed over his own spare tube and patch kit.

Ten minutes later, my front tire blew again. Unbelievable! Not once during my training had I suffered even two flats in a single ride. Witnessing my dismay, Craig popped his front wheel out of the fork, thrust it at me, and told me to keep moving while he repaired my wheel. I rode on for a few miles and then circled back. When my headlamp picked Craig out of the darkness, I saw that he was ready to go. We were now both out of spare tubes.

The sun rose, revealing a breathtaking view of the Pacific Ocean on one side of us and Kauai's majestic forests on the other. A helicopter appeared overhead and descended toward us. Craig let me ride ahead as the film crew captured aerial video. The chopper swung so low that locals came scrambling out of their houses to gawk. I wondered what our policeman friend would think.

I stopped at the precise point where my watch showed that I had completed 112 miles. But when I saved the ride file, the reading changed to 111.9 miles. So I got back on my bike and pedaled in circles for a tenth of a mile. There would be no rounding up in the Fifty.

Jordan, who now had the wheel of the van, chauffeured us back to the YMCA where I had begun my first of fifty triathlons at the stroke of midnight with a 170-lap swim in an outdoor pool, watched by a small gathering that included Sunny and our five pajama-clad children. By the time we got there, I was already wearing my running gear. Four of us—two more locals, Craig, and I—started the marathon together. We made our way east toward Lihue Airport in search of flatter roads to tread. Almost instantly, it seemed, it was eighty-four degrees and as humid as a jungle. I felt as though I were jogging through a simmering broth.

Running in Hawaii doesn't agree with me. I'd barfed my way through the Ironman World Championship marathon in Kona the previous year, and twenty miles into the first marathon of the Fifty I felt another purge coming. Lucky for me, the Divas and Dudes triathlon club joined me around halfway, and kept me running in the right direction, as I swallowed back the bile. The Cowboy 5k started in a hotel parking lot, where Lucy, Lily, and Daisy were excited to join me. We ran back toward the YMCA, all suffering from the heat and humidity. Daisy soon surrendered and hopped back into the car. By that point, the sickening sloshing of my stomach contents consumed my attention, and I was unable to engage with the twenty-plus people who had come out to run those last 3.1 miles with me. As we approached the YMCA for the last time, I turned to Craig. "I don't feel so well," I said.

The last quarter mile felt like a marathon in itself. When I stopped, a cheer went up. I darted to the side and dropped to all fours. A blast of foamy liquid shot out of my mouth with the force of a firehose. It went on forever. Stomach emptied, I slowly got to my feet and faced the crowd. The same people who had just been cheering for me now watched me in stunned silence. I drew the back of my hand across my mouth.

"One down, forty-nine to go," I said.

We landed in Anchorage at five o'clock the next morning. By five thirty, our ragtag party—Sunny, the kids, Jordan, the film crew, and me—was huddled at the curb outside baggage claim, woefully underdressed for the forty-eight-degree chill, burdened by enough luggage to support a small military campaign. At six o'clock, our rides still hadn't arrived. I was supposed to be swimming at seven.

At last, they came—my friend Bodie in an Isuzu Rodeo, and James, a friend of Jordan's father, in a pickup truck. Somehow all eleven of us squeezed into the two vehicles. We drove to James's house to unload our things and get prepared for the day. I then hopped in the truck, and we drove to the Alaska Club, which had opened early just for me. My local ambassador, Heather, awaited me there, ready to swim. Heather had reached out to me nine days earlier. She had shredded my plan for Day 2, telling me there were far better pools in Anchorage than the one I'd selected, that my bike route would have taken me over a 1,500-foot pass and that my marathon course was in an area where "people just don't run."

By nine o'clock, we were on our bikes, just the two of us, bundled against the cold in tights and arm sleeves. We rode southward from the city along the Seward Highway into postcard Alaska, skirting the icy waters of Turnagain Arm, creeping toward the snow-draped Chugach Mountains. I spotted a moose and stopped to photograph it. An eagle swooped down and glided behind us like a kite for several unreal minutes.

After two hours, I was over it, the natural splendor surrounding me rendered invisible by hunger. Before we'd left the club, Heather had asked me if I needed any nutritional support. I'd assured her my crew would take care of me. I had forgotten that I would not have my full crew until the next day, in Washington. As I spoke, the one crewman I did have, Jordan, was on his way back to James's house, where he would sleep for the next seven hours. I felt a very particular craving for a hot breakfast sandwich. Just then a familiar-looking Isuzu Rodeo pulled up next to us. The front passenger window opened, and Sunny's face appeared. "I've got a breakfast sandwich for you," she said.

Ninety minutes later, I was hungry again. Heather and I stopped at a gas station.

⑩ SO MUCH FOR THE PLAN

I picked out a bag of potato chips and a Monster energy drink and took them to the cash register. Only then did I remember I had no money.

"Don't worry about it," Heather said.

Our ride ended at Chain Reaction Cycles in South Anchorage, where I indulged in ninety seconds of interaction with Sunny and the kids. I had a dark intuition that this was how it was going to be every day. Heather and I changed into running gear and headed out on a bike path that hugged the main road for five miles and then diverged into parkland. We'd picked up one other companion at the store, Conway, a younger guy who told us he had never run farther than thirteen miles. I asked him how many miles he thought he had in him today, and he shrugged. I knew he was all in when he called his parents and asked them to bring food, which, when it arrived, I ate most of, Jordan having failed to appear.

"So what do you think?" Conway asked me some time later.

"Are you 100 percent positive that you're going to finish this thing, or are you just determined to do your best and see what happens?"

"I have to believe that I can do it," I said. "Otherwise, I wouldn't stand a chance."

We circled Westchester Lagoon, its surface gleaming like a freshly Windexed mirror, and then picked up the Tony Knowles Coastal Trail, which led us downtown to the meeting point for the Iron Cowboy 5K. A handful of local runners and triathletes, most of them friends of Heather, were there, as were Sunny and the kids and Conway's dad, Mitch, accompanied by what looked like a sled dog.

It turned out it *was* a sled dog. Not just any sled dog, but Wall-E, a member of the team that had won the previous year's Iditarod. Conway had been holding out on me. His father, I now learned, was a legendary musher and a two-time winner of the world's most prestigious sled dog race. Mitch strapped a belt around my waist and hitched a lead to Wall-E's harness. The dog then dragged me through the last few miles of my second triathlon, which sounds like cheating, but Wall-E wanted to go a lot faster than I did and I had to burn extra energy resisting him.

Upon reaching our stopping point, I was annoyed to discover that the film crew was nowhere to be seen. I called Jacob, the leader of the three-man team, and asked him where on earth he was. He asked me where on earth *I* was. We soon figured out that they had gone to the wrong park. While we waited for them to find us, I drank hot chicken broth from a thermos that Mitch had handed to me and signed the back of the bib that Conway had worn in the 5K: "Congratulations on your first marathon!"

When the film crew arrived, I cajoled Conway into rising stiff-legged from the curb and joining the rest of us in recreating the last fifty yards of the marathon for the camera's sake.

Never again would I voluntarily run farther than I had to.

The ruining of my right shoulder began at approximately 7:20 a.m. on Day 3, in Lake Stevens, fifty miles north of Seattle. Blind with fatigue (I had slept a cumulative nine hours in the past three nights on airplanes), I was failing miserably in my efforts to follow behind a kayaker. Aaron, who had driven up from Utah the day before with the rest of my crew, and my friend Carlee, were with me in the water as I felt a pinching kind of pain began deep inside my right shoulder. Having no option other than to continue swimming and hope the pain would go away, I did just that. Unsurprisingly, the pain did not go away, but only intensified as I swam crazy zigzags through the rippled water.

Back on shore, I went straight to Natalie, who had traveled there with the others, and asked her to work on the throbbing joint. She knelt with me for ten minutes outside the motor home, moving my right arm this way and that with one hand and digging into the shoulder with the other. I then went inside the RV to change into bike clothes and gather the supplies I would need for the next six and a half hours.

"Who's got my nutrition?" I asked Casey and Aaron.

They looked at each other, then back at me.

"Um, it's in the van," Casey said.

"And where's the van?" I asked.

"It's at the house," Aaron said.

The house that Aaron referred to was the Airbnb home Jordan had unaccountably booked forty-five minutes away from our current location. Sunny began rummaging through the RV's cramped kitchen in search of sustenance. Finding none, she rifled through the travel bags, eventually coming up with a Dr. Pepper, a small bag of nuts, and a single-serving packet of protein powder. To these items were added the energy bars and gels that Brittany, our friend, and Dallas' chiropractic assistant, had been planning to fuel herself with while riding with me.

We set off—Brittany, Carlee, me, and a couple of local supporters, one of whom—Christopher, a pastor, and triathlete—volunteered to guide us.

"Are we going to go this slow the whole way?" he asked after a few miles.

I stared at him for a moment before replying. "You do know I'm doing fifty of these things, right?" I said.

There were no further complaints about our tempo.

I had planned a two-loop bike route, but the back half of the loop proved to be a lot hillier than I'd anticipated, so I asked Christopher to lead us to flatter roads for our finish. We rolled back into the staging area at four thirty. I hastily changed into a speedo and jumped back in the lake to swim 259 yards. During the bike ride, David had sent me a text informing me I had not swum quite far enough. This was a consequence of my having forgotten to switch my watch from its pool setting to its open-water setting. The sleep deprivation was catching up to me. Twenty minutes later, I was dressed to run, minus my shoes.

"Who's got my shoes?" I asked.

Casey and Aaron looked at each other, then looked back at me.

"They're in the van," Casey confessed.

"How do you not have my shoes?" I fumed. "I hope everybody had a nice nap while I was out there getting my butt kicked!"

Sunny had already made one ninety-minute round-trip drive to the Airbnb house to collect my nutrition. She would now have to make a second one to deliver my running shoes. In the meantime, I took Casey's size elevens (I wear a twelve) and Casey took Aaron's size ten, so he could pace me through the first part of the marathon. Brittany, Carlee, and another handful of local supporters joined us.

As soon as I started running, an all-too-familiar soreness announced itself in my right hip. The same issue had dogged me throughout my world-record campaign in 2012. Less than three miles further on, the left side of my abdominal wall began to hurt. I had a history with this pain as well—it was the very one that had led me to Dallas, and that continued to bother me during my training for the Fifty.

Halfway through the marathon, we returned to the staging area, where I changed into my own shoes, ate, and got Natalie to work on my hip. We hit the trail again and almost immediately I was struck by what felt like a bad case of heartburn. What the heck was happening to my body? It seemed to be rapidly splitting apart along a jagged fault line running from pelvis to shoulder. I mentioned my newest complaint to Brittany, who suggested I call Dallas. We got him on the phone, and I described my symptoms.

"I think it's your hiatal hernia," he said, referring to yet another old ailment.

IRON COWBOY

"You probably aggravated it when you threw up in Hawaii."

The good news, he said, was that an adjustment ought to take care of it. The bad news was that Brittany had never performed the procedure, but she was game to try. I lay down on a patch of grass and Brittany squatted beside me. As my jogging companions looked on like so many surgical Internists, Dallas talked Brittany through the adjustment on speakerphone. From my perspective, she seemed to be trying to reach through my intestines and grab my spine. After a few unpleasant minutes, we stood up and set off again. I could tell that Brittany was waiting for me to say how much better I felt, but my silent grimace said something else.

"Let's try it again," she said.

"Forget it," I said. "It's a waste of time."

Brittany persisted, I relented, and we got back on the ground. This time I felt a sudden, gushy release, like a finger coming unstuck from a bottleneck, except the finger was my esophagus, and the bottle was my stomach. I now could worry about one less sore spot.

By this point, we had picked up a young Japanese-American man whose lakeside home we had run past just as he was backing out of his driveway to search for us. I noticed right away that his legs were covered in old scars and there was a hitch in his stride. Curious, I asked to hear his story. "I got run over by a bus," he said.

Ten years earlier, when Keito was sixteen years old, a full-size school bus had squashed him on his way to school. He spent the next five weeks in the hospital and went home in a wheelchair. When he was able to walk again, Keito rejoined his high school swim team. Unable to match his former times, he grew frustrated and quit. He lost most of the next decade to depression. Eventually, Keito sought counseling, which helped a little, and then he started running, which helped a lot. He told me he'd never run farther than six miles, but would try for ten. When he got to ten miles—which was sixteen miles for me—he kept going.

"Do you think I could do an Ironman?" Keito asked me.

"It doesn't matter what I think," I said. "If *you* believe you can do it, then I'll guarantee you can."

Keito ran twenty miles with me, all the way to the finish line of my third of fifty triathlons. No sooner had I released him from a bear hug than he collapsed to the ground. Unable to get up by his own power, he was lifted into the back of the Subaru and driven home by Casey and Aaron. The next day, Keito registered for an Ironman.

⑩ SO MUCH FOR THE PLAN

I pedaled away from Clackamas Cove the next morning with a worsened right shoulder and a single companion, Dean, a friend of my Oregon ambassador, Carmen. As Dean and I crept northward along stoplight-infested urban roads toward the Portland waterfront, Carmen drove ahead to meet us at various checkpoints, ringing a cowbell at each of them so we wouldn't miss her. Our third stop came at thirty-four miles.

"I'm starving," I announced as we rolled in. "I need you to get me some food."

My manners had left me a couple of states back. Carmen didn't seem to mind. With a proud smile and not a word was spoken, she handed over a hot breakfast burrito and a scone.

"Thanks," I said. "But I'd also like a sandwich, a bag of chips, and a Monster energy drink."

Carmen promised to have these things waiting for me at the next checkpoint. Soon after I wheeled away, I developed tunnel vision, the world contracting to a narrow cone of light and color in front of me. When a supporter to my left or right spoke, the voice came from nowhere. I spoke little, and when I did, I could barely hear myself. Suddenly my head snapped up. I had nodded off for a split second, a primal reflex saving me from catastrophe. I willed myself to stay alert, but my sleepiness had an irresistible magnetism, and I lost consciousness twice more before reaching the next checkpoint.

A former surgical technician, Carmen took one look at me and gently pulled me off my bike. I offered no resistance. She opened the driver door of her car and chivvied me inside, reclined the seat, unzipped my jersey, and wrapped my hand around the energy drink she'd bought for me. I passed out instantly. After just five minutes Carmen woke me again, knowing I was already at some risk of missing my eight forty-five p.m. flight to San Jose. I felt remarkably refreshed.

Exactly seven hours before my boarding time, I left the New Seasons Market parking lot on foot to begin my marathon with a picturesque two-loop jaunt along the waterfront. There was little fanfare, actually none. But when I came back four hours and twenty-five minutes later for the Iron Cowboy 5K, the place had become a hive of activity. A crowd of thirty or more Oregonians dressed to run in ninety-degree heat milled about the motor home. My sister Sandra, and her husband Andrew, happened to be in town visiting friends. They too came to run the 5k. Lucy and Lily were flitting among the crowd, distributing number bibs and safety pins. Sunny was visiting with supporters and taking donations to the Jamie Oliver Food Foundation. The store's management had set up a booth and tables, from which aproned employees handed out protein bars and chunks of fresh watermelon. There was a reporter for KATU television there to capture it all.

A lump of emotion lodged in my throat as I took it all in. Here were the first small signs that my vision for this crazy endeavor might be realized in some meaningful way—that the Fifty would be something more than an endorphin junkie's self-indulgence.

I guzzled a Cosmic Cranberry Kombucha, placed a ridiculous red-and-white-striped cowboy hat atop my head, and led the crowd out for the 5K. When I finished, I wrapped my arms around Carmen, lifted her, and whirled her in a circle, punch-drunk. Back on her feet, Carmen grabbed a microphone and said a few words before inviting me to speak.

"I just want to thank everyone for coming out," I said. "This is a huge journey for my family and me."

My vision swam. I put a fist to my lips to suppress a sob, then dropped my chin to signal *give me a minute*. An embarrassed hush fell upon the group. Quinn broke from Sunny's side and ran to me. I lifted him, and he wrapped his legs around my waist like a baby chimp. One or two women in the crowd said "Aw," eliciting titters that lightened the moment. Even then, I couldn't get out much more besides, "Thank you, Oregon."

I landed in San Jose at ten thirty that night, only three hours after completing triathlon number four, having *barely* made my flight from Portland. Aaron and Natalie were waiting for me at the curb in the Subaru. My backup bicycle, which I had never ridden, was secured to the roof. They had left Portland around the time I was eating the breakfast burrito Carmen bought me and arrived at the airport minutes ahead of me. The others would drive through the night and, with any luck, would reach Santa Cruz, the site of my next triathlon, in time to see me wade out of the Pacific Ocean tomorrow morning. I had to force myself not to visualize Casey hunkering red-eyed over the RV's giant steering wheel with all that precious human cargo behind him.

Aaron, zombified from his own lack of sleep, could not find the house in Santa Cruz we'd rented through Airbnb. In the end, I was forced to wake the owner with a phone call and have him guide us in. There was one bed available and, of course, it was all mine. I flopped onto the queen-size pillow-top mattress and let out a groan of ecstasy. Never again would I take such simple comforts for granted.

Natalie asked if there were specific parts of my body that needed particular attention. I pointed to a pair of fresh, fluid-filled blisters on my left foot and asked her to pop them.

"Ew, gross!" she said. "That's not even in my job description. Anyway, I don't think it's a good idea."

"I think it's a great idea," I said. "Please?"

Natalie caved and did the grody deed, then massaged my muscles for a couple of hours while I slept. When she shook me awake at six o'clock a.m., I was in the exact same position that she had last seen me. Aaron, Natalie, and I climbed inside the Subaru and made the short drive to Cowell Beach on Monterey Bay. Having failed to recruit a California state ambassador, I didn't expect to find anyone waiting for us there; to my surprise, we were greeted by a group of eight to ten supporters.

I squeezed into my wetsuit and splashed into the frigid ocean with a lack of hesitation that belied my inner reluctance. The first stinging contact between my blistered left foot and the sixty-degree brine made me regret my insistence on the previous night's lancing. This bit of discomfort was quickly displaced, however, by the agony in my right shoulder as I struggled through thick kelp along Santa Cruz Wharf with three other swimmers. I pictured muscle tearing away from the bone like rib meat in a dog's jaws.

I completed half the swim and hauled myself back onto the beach, where Natalie worked on the shoulder before a mute audience, my teeth clacking as she poked and pressed ineffectually through my neoprene second skin. After the second loop, Natalie took me by a shivering arm and led me to a cold outdoor shower to wash the sand out of my blisters. A steaming bowl of steel-cut oats brought to me by a supporter, from a café across the street, began the long process of restoring my body's temperature equilibrium.

An 112-mile bike ride completed it. Steve, the president of the local triathlon club, guided a handful of local supporters and me out of the parking lot and onto Highway 101 North. We'd gone no farther than three or four miles when I heard a honk and saw the Iron Cowboy motor home pass. I saw everyone waving their hands excitedly and heard them cheer out of open windows. I felt my whole body relax.

My intention had been to ride all the way to Half Moon Bay and back. But at forty miles, just past Pescadero, we hit a steep climb, and my heart rate spiked unacceptably. I turned to Steve. "I can't do this," I said. "Can you take me somewhere flatter?"

And so it was that, for the fifth time in as many days, I abandoned a bike course I had spent hours planning out over the winter.

On the way back to Santa Cruz, we were joined by a man who appeared to weigh more than 300 pounds, named Joe. Having driven down from San Francisco to see me, Joe eagerly placed himself at the front of our group, which now numbered eleven, joking that his wide body would create a slipstream for all of us. Within minutes, he was hanging on to the rear of the paceline, gasping. A half hour later, he was gone.

As brief as his involvement in the campaign was, Joe took something away from it. Each day after that, he made sure to ride ten to twelve miles, calling it "my 10 percent" because it was 10 percent as far as I was riding each day. Over the next few months, he lost forty-five pounds.

At three thirty in the afternoon, a local athlete hopped on a mountain bike and led me out onto the marathon course with a fresh batch of supporters. We headed north along a bluff that offered a panoramic view of the sun-dappled ocean below. A salt-scented onshore breeze refreshed us, as if by friendly intent. Seagulls wheeled and screeched overhead, and I couldn't help but think how classically Californian the moment was.

We returned to the staging area to find the parking lot bustling with people ready to run the Iron Cowboy 5K with me, perhaps fifty in all. That was the good news. The bad news was that Casey and Aaron had no idea what to do with them. Apparently, they had just discovered our lack of a local ambassador and learned that no route had been chosen for the 5K. They were now running around in a dither, trying to find someone to volunteer for the role.

Of greater concern to me was the fact that I had fallen more than an hour behind schedule. My next triathlon was supposed to start 535 miles away in Las Vegas in a little more than twelve hours. Realizing I couldn't possibly reach my destination in time to start Day 6 on time traveling in the motor home, I asked Aaron to fix up a sleeping pallet for me in the Subaru and to pack a bag with the stuff I'd need in the morning. The much roomier van was not an option because it was crammed top to bottom with unopened boxes of Iron Cowboy giveaways—hats, T-shirts, sunglasses, running shoes, earbuds, and more—that the crew hadn't gotten around to giving away yet. We were not firing on all cylinders.

It was nearing ten o'clock at night, when I said goodbye to my last lingering supporter, I sat down on the entry step of the motor home in an emptied-out parking lot, and began sipping from a carton of coconut water. Julie, a reporter for the *Santa Cruz Sentinel,* stood over me and asked about my recently completed triathlon. The day had come full circle. Thirteen hours earlier, Julie had stood over me while I trembled under an icy foot bath, ate oatmeal left-handed, and looked with consternation at the sand-encrusted blisters on my right foot.

"How's it going so far?" she'd asked.

"It's not off to a very good start, I'm afraid," I said.

I was talking about Day 5, of course, not about the campaign as a whole.

I sincerely hoped.

⑪
PLAYING KETCHUP
DAYS 27–28
MARYLAND, DELAWARE

A chirping cell phone alarm woke Casey and Aaron at six o'clock in the morning on Day 27. They threw on shorts and T-shirts and fumbled their way out of the RV and onto the parking lot at Great Marsh Park, a grassy riverside recreational area in Cambridge, Maryland, expecting to find the van parked nearby. It was not. They texted Jordan, who was delivering me from Morgantown, asking where the heck he was. No response.

Where's Jordan? This question had become a bitter running joke within Team Iron Cowboy. My project manager had a penchant for absconding with the van when it was needed and for going incommunicado when *he* was needed. But this was the first time he had disappeared *with me.*

An hour passed. It was now seven o'clock, and I was supposed to be in the Choptank River. The wingmen made repeated apologies to Jason, my Maryland ambassador, who'd been up since four and on-site since five thirty. Another hour passed. Casey and Aaron—who don't freak out easily—began to freak out.

It was past eight thirty when the van finally rolled in. The reason for our late arrival was simple: My trip to Haydn's hotel room for a late-night massage the night before had set us back. I have no explanation, however, for Jordan's radio silence. I was asleep.

The wingmen flung open the van's side door and presented me with a bowl of quinoa oatmeal and a salad of organic greens and chicken. I sat with my back against the interior wall, eating and slowly coming around as Sunny massaged my feet. A man with a gray mustache and matching soul patch approached and introduced himself as Paul, a reporter for the *Dorchester Banner.* I decided to have a little fun with him.

"You get two questions," I said, "and they both have to be original. You have to ask me something I haven't been asked before."

Paul looked pensive, obviously willing to play along.

"I've got something," he said brightly. "What do you think of the idea of putting Harriet Tubman on the ten-dollar bill?"

I stopped chewing mid-mouthful. "That was a good one," I said. "You can ask me anything you want now."

"Do you still think this is a good idea?" Paul asked. "Do you still have a full heart for the project?"

This question gave me pause in a different way. Just eight hours earlier, after completing my triathlon in West Virginia, I had texted David, expressing serious doubts that everything I was going through, and putting Sunny and the crew through, would turn out to be worthwhile. David had assured me it would.

"Oh, I still think it's a great idea," I said to Paul. "I've got a ton of support. When you see donations coming in, and when you see that you're making a difference, how can that be a bad idea?"

The truth was that our fund-raising thus far had been more than a little disappointing to me. I had vowed to raise one million dollars to fight childhood obesity, but we'd brought in less than $20,000 to date. They say all press is good press, but the hammering I was taking online from my haters seemed to have made a lot of the Fifty's followers hesitant to support my cause. Yet, I still felt I was making a difference, albeit one person at a time, through my encounters with people like Keito in Washington and Valerie in Maryland. The good you do is not always the good you expected to do.

As the wingmen hustled me from the van to the motor home to get ready to swim, I caught a glimpse of the river. A stiff wind had stirred the slate-gray water into a forbidding chop. Dark clouds hung close to the surface, reducing visibility to near zero, and the western sky looked threatening. When the rain started, I sent Casey back outside to fetch Jason.

"What's the weather report?" I asked him.

"It's supposed to clear up later," he said.

"How much later?" I asked.

⑪ PLAYING KETCHUP

"A lot later," he admitted.

Already hours behind schedule, I couldn't afford to wait hours more to start swimming.

"What's plan B?" I asked.

Within fifteen minutes I was standing on the deck of a six-lane indoor pool at a nearby YMCA, poised to execute my patented sideways fall into the water. Just then a thunderclap sounded in the near distance. A lifeguard stepped forward and waved her arms.

"Everyone out of the pool!" she shouted.

I turned to Jason with palms upturned. *What gives?*

"There's a law in Maryland," he said. "No swimming—not even indoors—until thirty minutes after the thunder stops."

I found a bench to sit on, while the thunder kept coming. I told myself not to waste mental energy worrying about something I couldn't control, but every now and again I caught myself rocking to and fro, itching to get moving.

At last, there came a break in the thunder. I got up and approached Jason.

"Has it been thirty minutes?" I asked, knowing it hadn't. "Do you think they'll let me in a little early?"

Jason was just opening his mouth to reply when another rumble reached our ears. The clock went back to zero.

I sat down again. The sky kept booming. After a few minutes, I got up and approached Jason a second time.

"Isn't there someone you can talk to?" I asked. "I'm willing to sign a waiver. Whatever it takes."

It was now ten o'clock, far later than I'd started any of my twenty-six previous triathlons. If I lost another hour, I might lose an entire day, and the campaign would be totally sunk. Fifty triathlons in fifty states in fifty-*one* days just doesn't have the same ring to it.

Jason told me that, in fact, there was somebody he could try to talk to, Gary, the president of the Dorchester County YMCA's board of directors and a triathlete himself. Minutes later, Gary arrived in the flesh, accompanied by the facility's CEO, JoAnn. They'd been meeting in Gary's office when Jason's urgent text message came through. The two executives huddled with Jason and Barbara, the lifeguard who'd put the kybosh on my swim start. They spoke in low voices and then beckoned to me.

"We'll let you swim," Gary said. "But you're the only one allowed in the pool. And we *do* want you to sign a waiver."

"Oh, thank you! Thank you!" I gushed. "You can have one of my kids. They're right outside in the RV."

Without further delay, I entered the water, an audience of more than twenty envious would-be swimmers looking on. I stroked across the pool and back, then stopped.

"One!" I called out.

I completed the remaining 83.5 laps as quickly as I could, but I was unable to make up any time because of the sorry state of my right shoulder. At eleven thirty, I left the water knowing that I would have to take some risks on the bike. Luckily, Jason had chosen the official Ironman Maryland bike course as my cycling route, and it was dead flat. After a hasty costume change, I sank my sore rear end onto the saddle and started to grind. Within a few miles, people were popping off the back of our group. Paul, the reporter who had interviewed me earlier, followed behind our human-powered freight train in his car, clocking us at twenty-five miles per hour at one point.

Jason had recruited a physician, a chiropractor, and a massage therapist to attend to my needs between the bike ride and the marathon, but I passed on all three of them, taking a gamble with my health for the sake of time. He showed up for the 5K riding a hybrid mountain bike and towing a baby trailer packed with food and drinks. I laughed.

"Go ahead and laugh," Jason said, "but in about fifteen miles you're going to love this thing."

We ran northward along the river to Hambrooke Point and back—1.55 miles each way. It was a gorgeously scenic place to work up a sweat, with smooth, silent water on one side and lush greenery on the other.

"I just want to keep doing this," I told Jason.

Jason couldn't hide his disappointment—he had wanted me to follow the run course of the Ironman 70.3 Eagleman, a race he coordinated—but he politely agreed to my proposal. After a couple more laps, however, he talked me into extending our route another mile, to Long Wharf Park, for variety's sake.

Around sunset, I felt a major bonk coming on. I fought the fatigue as best I could by eating huge numbers of homemade rice bars that Jason's wife, Laura, had baked for me and requested that Jason remind me to drink every fifteen minutes. At one point he caught me eyeing the bottle of lemonade, he was sipping from, and he handed it over without a word. I finished it in one long swig.

Still dragging—and still hungry—I asked Jason to stop his bike, so I could grab a sandwich he had bought earlier at a convenience store and stashed in the baby trailer. (He'd been right, after all. I did love it now!) I tore the wrapper off, handed one-half of the foot-long hoagie to Jason to save for me, and started running with the other half. I took a big bite and nearly spit it out, tasting hot peppers and oil.

"I can't eat this!" I complained. "It'll tear me up."

"Great, because it's not yours," Jason said. "It's mine. I got plain turkey and veggies for you."

As the hours passed, my weariness deepened. My running companions knew I was in trouble when I stopped talking altogether. Eventually, they too fell silent.

"I'm in a dark place," I confessed to Jason.

"There's nothing I can tell you that you can't tell yourself to get through this," he said. "I'm pretty sure you know every mental trick in the book."

He was right again. As wretched as I was feeling, a part of me was also rejoicing because in my entire life as a triathlete, *I had never had two bad days in a row.* And so while I couldn't wait for this day to be over, I also couldn't wait for tomorrow to begin. All I had to do was make it there.

One of my running companions was Paul, a lifelong couch potato who had weighed 300 pounds before he recently took up triathlon and became a vegan. At sixteen miles, we took a break so I could loosen up my legs with a self-massage stick. Paul looked at his watch and said something I didn't quite catch. Another person repeated it, but again I missed the words.

"What is it? What's going on?" I asked.

"I just realized that I've run farther than I've ever run before," Paul said.

I tossed the massage stick aside theatrically and started a slow clap, like in the movies. The others joined in. (They must have seen the same films.) We clapped louder and faster as Paul smiled and blushed. The only thing missing was sappy music, heavy on the strings. Even in the midst of my own journey, I was proud of Paul, and it was important to me to celebrate this moment with him.

When we returned to Great Marsh Park, I had one-sixth of a mile left to cover. I had never been more tempted to call it "close enough," but I bit the bullet and finished off triathlon number twenty-seven with four grim laps around the park. Jordan crawled out of the van to take the customary finish photos. After everyone else had left, he snapped one more picture. Time-stamped at 12:36 a.m., it shows me sitting on a step outside the door of the motor home with my elbows on my knees and my head hanging.

No doubt about it: tomorrow was going to be terrific.

While I was running late—literally and figuratively—in Maryland, my friend Dano in Utah was on the phone with my Delaware ambassador, Laura, asking her to do everything in her power to get me back on schedule on Day 28. Laura took this appeal seriously—very seriously.

No sooner had the wingmen popped their heads out of the RV at the Dover YMCA than Laura collared them and insisted they rouse me right away and get me going. Cowed by her schoolmarm manner, Casey and Aaron did as they were instructed. At seven o'clock sharp, I toppled sideways into the Y's outdoor pool. A dozen locals, including Laura, swam with me, as did Sunny and the wingmen.

As usual, my wife and friends quickly lost interest in churning out laps and started acting foolish—splashing and dunking each other and screeching like five-year-olds. At one point, Laura came to the wall when the four of us were standing there laughing at something silly that Casey had done. She stopped and raised her goggles to her forehead.

"You might not take these swims very seriously," she snapped, "but I have a workout to get done!"

We laughed even harder.

After I'd completed my swim, Laura pulled me aside. I thought I was going to get another scolding.

"I'm sorry I was so grumpy earlier," she said matter-of-factly, "I just want everything to go right today."

"Please, don't apologize," I said. "We're all grateful for everything you're doing. We need someone to crack the whip sometimes."

As I spoke to her, I sensed Laura had been through a tough experience of some kind that had tainted her natural warmth with a flinty toughness. I would eventually learn from Laura herself that this was indeed the case. In 1998, when she was thirty-five, Laura was diagnosed with breast cancer. Few families have been ravaged by this disease more ruthlessly than hers. Lung cancer killed Laura's mother, ovarian cancer

⑪ PLAYING KETCHUP

took her older sister, and two other siblings fought and beat the big *C*. Laura survived as well, but her battle with cancer left her scarred both physically and emotionally, and it took her years to recover from the effects of chemotherapy. In the meantime, her first and second marriages unraveled and she resorted to alcohol to cope.

Things began to turn around for Laura when she joined a gym in Milwaukee, where she was then living, and began to work out with a group of other recently sedentary women. One of these workout buddies talked her into running a half marathon. Crossing that first finish line made Laura feel whole again for the first time since her diagnosis. It also made her hungry for more, and other finish lines followed, each one energizing her a little more.

"I am not simply surviving; I am living," Laura told a reporter in 2011 while training for her first Ironman at age fifty, and in the process raising nearly $5,000 to combat breast cancer. "I have found a way to give back. I continue to share my story and to add new chapters. Breast cancer may win some battles, but it doesn't have to win the game. The fire that has been unleashed in my belly to fight, for others and myself, is something that the disease cannot take away."

Now that's my kind of gal.

A local bike shop owner, Dave, and his wife, Cecilia, brought breakfast. They laid down trays of scrambled eggs and hash browns on the outdoor table where I was seated, then set it with paper plates and plastic forks. Given the quantities I'd asked them to prepare, they'd naturally assumed the food was intended to feed my whole family. Dave's eyebrows lifted and Cecilia's jaw went slack when I grabbed both trays of food and placed them on my lap.

"Got any ketchup?" I asked.

Someone produced a bottle of Heinz. I turned it upside down and squeezed half its contents onto the potatoes, the other half onto the eggs, picked up a fork, and dug in. I could not lift the fork to my face, however. My right shoulder hurt so much, especially after swimming, that I had to bring my face to the fork, like an ape. I was now one step away from belonging in a cage.

"Glad you like my cooking," Cecilia joked.

When the trays had been emptied of every last morsel, two local triathlon coaches, Jim and Anna, stepped forward and offered to guide me on their bikes from my present location to Fifer Orchards, our staging area for the rest of the day. Fifer is a fourth-generation family farm that started in 1919 by the great-grandfather of its current operator, a guy named Mike. Knowing little about triathlon, Mike had struggled to understand the scope of my undertaking when Laura approached him months earlier to propose that he host the bike ride and run portions of my day in Delaware.

"Put it this way," she'd told him. "I doubt James will even make it this far. You probably won't have to do anything."

A large gathering of cyclists—perhaps sixty—met me at the farm. Jim then led us around a thirteen-mile circuit that, to my satisfaction, not only was flat and quiet but included no left turns across traffic lanes and not a single stop sign. It's only negative was the occasional mound of horse poop to watch out for, left by horses, which belonged to the area's many Amish people.

While I rode, my family got to see another side of the local culture. The area's leading pastor, Rick, and his wife, Kari, and several of their ten children had come to the YMCA to watch me swim. They had learned about my mission from Savannah, their eldest daughter, who held a summer job at Fifer Orchards. As the mother of a large family, Kari could imagine better than most what Sunny was going through on this journey, so she approached her at poolside and offered up her hospitality. Sunny asked if she could do laundry, "Of course, we have two washers and dryers." This news was magic to Sunny's ears!

Pastor Rick's family was remarkably generous, opening their home to Sunny and the crew for the day. They were a simple Christian family, homeschooling their children, devoting time to their faith, and content with a simple life. The younger boys and girls dropped their jaws in awe when they saw the motorhome. My kids asked permission to show their new friends inside. This tour extended to them playing in the motorhome for several hours. It was an afternoon that all of the kids would remember, playing house, hide and seek, and enjoying the toys that they had acquired throughout our journey.

After lunch, Sunny and the kids came to the orchard, where Mike took them blueberry picking. By then I was making my final circuit of the bike course. Midway through it, I punctured a tire. I'd almost known it was coming, like a second sneeze after the first. Throughout the Fifty, flat tires had come in bunches. I would go days without experiencing any and then get three in a single ride. Today's first flat tire had occurred at ten miles. A local supporter, Suzanne, had loaned me a wheel from her bike so I could keep going.

This time it was Aaron who gave up a wheel and who, just as Suzanne had done earlier, sat down at the roadside to await rescue from Dave. As I pedaled away, it

⑪ PLAYING KETCHUP

occurred to me that I had been spoiled on the Fifty. Any child, who was treated by his or her parents the way *everyone* was treating me, would most surely grow up to become a monster of self-entitlement.

Approaching the farm, I heard music. It was Dave's daughter Emily, a singer-songwriter, who crooned in a smooth voice while accompanying herself on acoustic guitar. She had an appreciative audience in the healthy gathering of Delawareans who had come out for the Iron Cowboy 5K. Some were relaxing in the shade of walnut trees, others buying T-shirts and receiving race numbers from my kids. All were smiling. And why not? It was the first Saturday in July, seventy-five degrees and clear-skied. Sunny would tell me later it was the first day of our tour that felt almost normal—like summer at home.

It was with a large relief that I removed my derriere, now sore to the point of distraction, from my bike seat. Laura asked me if I wanted a massage, having lined up a local masseuse for me, but I declined, still anxious about time. So she led me directly to the farm store—a healthy eater's paradise of fresh produce, gourmet preserves, and organic everything—which had a small bathroom at the back where I could change into running clothes. Aaron stood guard outside the door. When Mike came upon him there, he invited us up to his house to freshen up and grab a snack.

"Is there any particular kind of fruit you'd like?" Mike asked as we walked.

"Watermelon," I said.

The stuff I'd eaten earlier in the day, blood red and intensely flavorful, had ruined me for any other watermelon I would eat.

"I'll cut one up for you," Mike said.

"I've also heard you guys make some amazing peach ice cream," I said leadingly.

"That we do," Mike said. "I'll have some ready to take with you tonight."

"Can I have it now?" I asked.

"You mean you're going to eat ice cream before you run a marathon?" Mike asked.

"Is that weird?" I joked.

Mike asked us to take a seat on a sofa in the front room, then disappeared into the kitchen. He came back with half a watermelon, halved lengthwise, a pint of ice cream, a spoon, and a Fifer Orchards trucker hat, which he casually dropped on the cushion next to me. I ate the entire half watermelon and the full pint of ice cream with the same spoon. As I rose to go and start my marathon, I grabbed the trucker hat—which was not the kind of hat anybody runs in—and plunked it on my head.

IRON COWBOY

After the 5K, my support shrank to the usual handful of endurance warriors willing and able to see me to the finish line. Among them was Le, a bespectacled Asian man who held a high-paying job in the financial services industry and had driven down from Wilmington early in the morning in a shiny black Porsche. He had swum the full 2.4 miles with me at the Dover YMCA, had followed my wheel for 112 miles on the bike, and was now close to finishing the marathon, despite never having run a marathon before, let alone done an Ironman. Before the 5K, Le had borrowed ten dollars from a stranger to purchase an Iron Cowboy T-shirt; he hadn't brought any cash. He didn't talk much, but I got the feeling this day was important to him.

With a few miles left, I became acutely sensitive to the backdrop to our small group's soft conversation, as I sometimes did in the waning moments of a day's triathlon. An almost full moon loomed above us, partly obscured by shadowy whips of clouds. Millions of crickets wove a high-pitched sonic tapestry with their insect voices. The air was country fresh, carrying just a whiff of horse poop.

"Everyone stop talking," I announced.

Everyone stopped talking. We glided along for a few dozen paces in companionable silence, seeing the moon, hearing the crickets, tasting the air.

"This is one of those moments," I said. "Just take it in. You'll remember it for the rest of your life."

Le's ejection soon broke the spell I was in, gazing into the sky. He was finally struggling. Turning around, I saw his features twisted in pain. I faced forward again and pressed on toward Fifer Orchards with the others, hoping Le would find within himself whatever he needed to survive just a few minutes longer.

Laura stood waiting at the finish. She held her arms wide to receive me, and I ran straight into her embrace.

"This is my favorite hug ever," she said.

When at last Laura let go, I turned back in the direction from where I had just come. Before long I spotted Le's reflective vest in the distance. When he saw us, he got up on his toes and sprinted the last twenty-five yards. Then it was our turn to embrace. One look into his eyes confirmed my earlier impression about what this day meant to him.

Mike, too, was present, having stayed up well past his farmer's bedtime to bear witness.

"What else can we do for you?" he asked.

⑪ PLAYING KETCHUP

"I'd really like a shower," I said.

He led me back to the house, Aaron again tagging along. This time, though, we entered not into the primary structure, but a smaller addition that had been built for Mike's grandmother, who had passed away a few years before at age ninety-one. We came to the foot of a wooden staircase.

"Bathroom's upstairs on the right," Mike said. "You'll find clean towels in there."

But I wasn't paying attention. My gaze was rooted on what appeared to be a stair lift—one of those sideways-facing, electric-powered chairs that glides up and down stairs.

"Does that thing work?" I asked.

"I think so," Mike said.

"Can I use it?"

"I don't see why not," Mike chuckled.

He folded the seat down and gestured for me to sit. I placed my feet on the footrest and discovered a seatbelt, which I promptly fastened. Mike flipped a switch, and I began to rise incredibly slowly. Aaron, of course, whipped out his phone and snapped a photo for social media.

Freshly scrubbed and cleanly dressed, I rode the chair lift back down to the ground floor. Mike and Aaron heard the electric motor whirring and burst out laughing.

I was hungry again—and I had a particular craving, as I so often did.

"Do we have any cereal?" I asked Aaron.

"Yeah, but we don't have milk."

"How can we have cereal and no milk?" I asked.

"Because the refrigerator isn't working," Aaron said.

"Why isn't the refrigerator working?"

"The refrigerator only worked for the first couple of days."

"Really?" I said. "Is the generator on?"

"The generator hasn't been working for ten days, that's why there is no air conditioner," Aaron responded.

Nothing in the RV, it seemed, was working. At this point, I gave myself better odds of making it to Utah than I did our Fleetwood Storm.

"I've got milk in the main house," Mike said.

We left Fifer Orchards just before midnight. The drive to Sea Bright, New Jersey, would take less than three hours. We were back on track.

IRON COWBOY

PHOTO COLLAGE

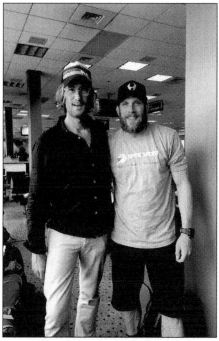

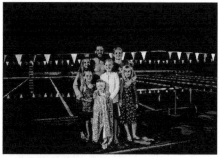

It all started poolside in Hawaii.

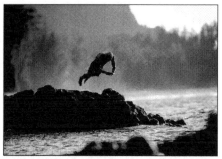

Ran into Rich Roll at the SLC airport.

Messing around in Hawaii.

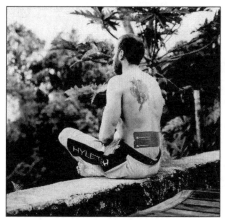

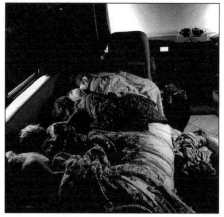

Meditating in Hawaii before day #1.

My five children sound asleep in the RV.

IRON COWBOY

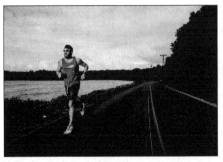
Run photo shoot in Hawaii.

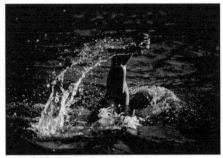
Swim prep in Hawaii prior to the start.

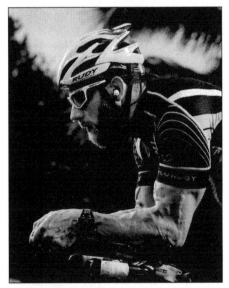
Pre 50 prep ride in Hawaii.

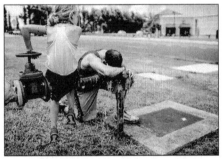
Sick as a dog post marathon #1 in Hawaii.

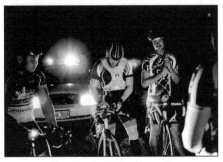
Twenty miles into the bike, the police stopped us.

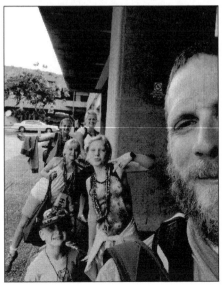
At the airport after Ironman #1 in Hawaii.

PHOTO COLLAGE

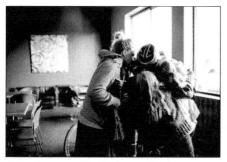

A much needed family hug in Alaska.

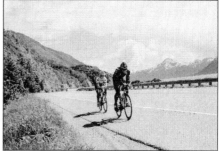

One of my favorite bike rides was in Alaska.

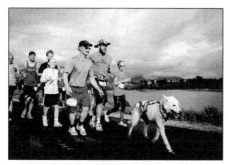

Run to the finish with the champion dogs in Alaska.

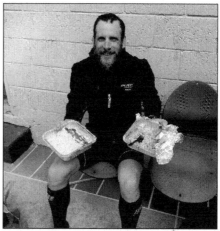

Eggs and potatoes were a staple breakfast for me.

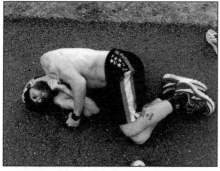

Early diaphragm struggles on day #3 in Washington.

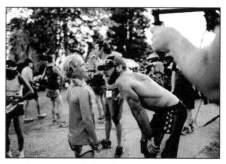

Lily doing her third 5k in a row with me in Washington.

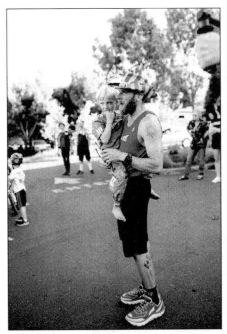

Pre 5k speech in Oregon with Quinn.

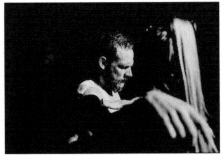

Getting worked on by natalie with the first signs of shoulder issues.

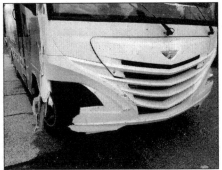

The poor RV after Casey hits a deer en route to Arizona.

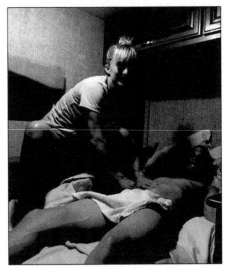

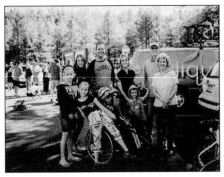

Dayton and his family in Arizona.

Getting worked on by Natalie with the first signs of shoulder issues.

PHOTO COLLAGE

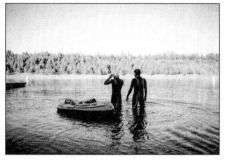

Morning swim with Dayton and Casey.

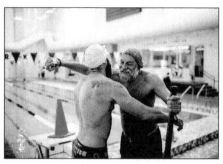

Swimming with friends in Nevada.

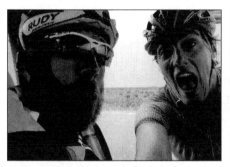

Sonja and I getting caught in the rain in Colorado.

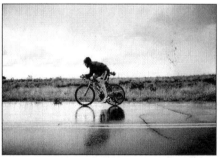

Cold wet ride in Colorado.

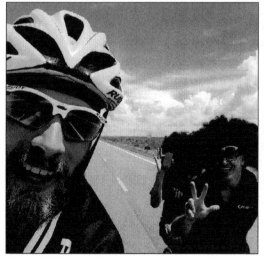

Eric and his son making me smile in Colorado on day #8.

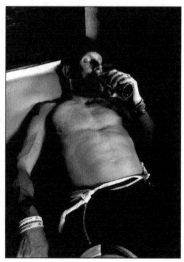

Falling asleep everywhere.

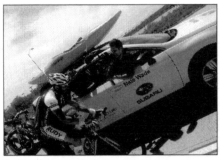

Rudy Project doing some filming.

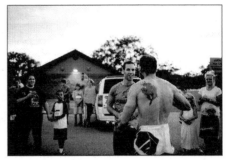

The gift of the US flag is one I will cherish forever.

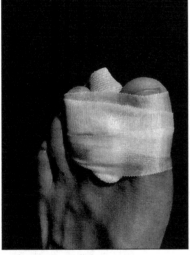

Trying to fix my feet.

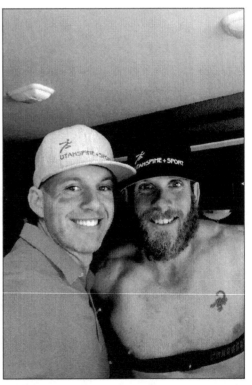

My close friend, Dr. Dallas Makin.

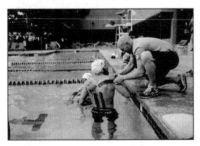

Dr. Dallas to the rescue pool side after tearing my shoulder.

PHOTO COLLAGE

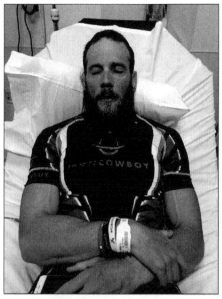

Blood work in Kansas.

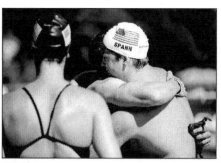

Getting some energy from Spann after my swim.

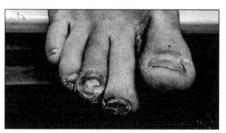

My foot, early in the journey.

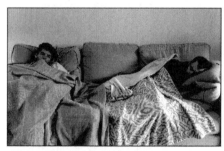

Casey and Aaron resting in Louisiana.

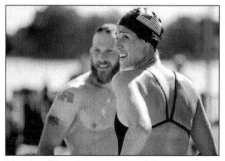

Meeting Olympians was special on this journey.

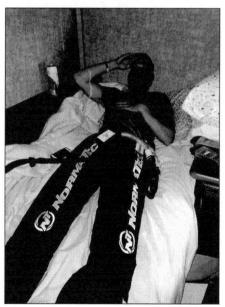

NormaTec session en route to the next State.

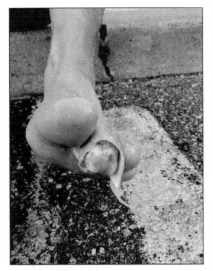

Mangled digit in Kentucky.

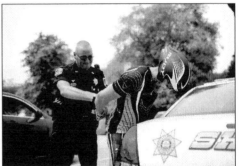

Having some fun Lieutenant Starnes.

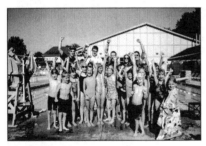

Humbled with everyone that came out to support.

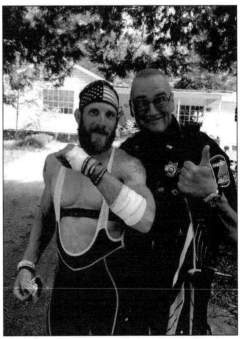

All fixed with Lieutenant Starnes.

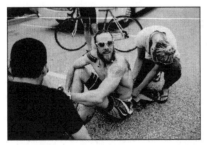

I never knew what transitions would look like.

PHOTO COLLAGE

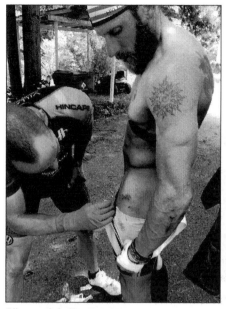

Bike crash in Tennessee.

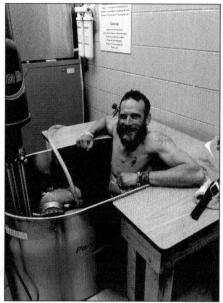

Post marathon ice bath in Tennessee.

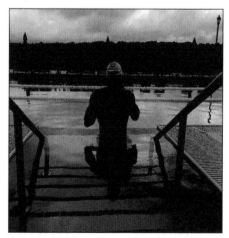

Contemplating the swim in Alabama.

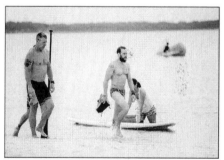

Swim done in Florida.

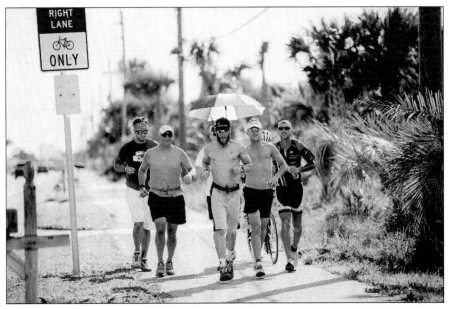

It is hot in Florida.

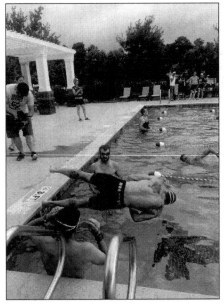

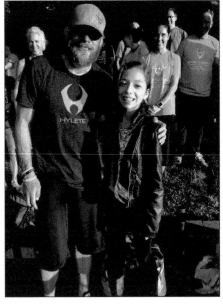

Smooth pool entry in South Carolina.   Beautiful anthem sang in North Carolina.

PHOTO COLLAGE

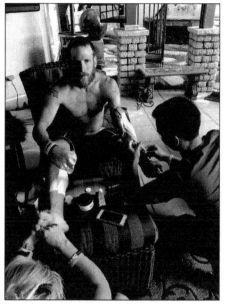

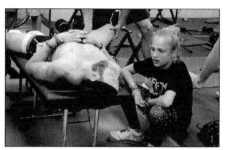

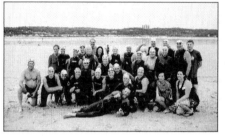

Reconnecting with Lucy in North Carolina.

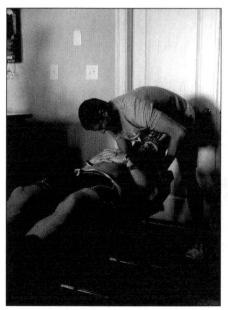

Drug testing in North Carolina.

Swim start in New Jersey.

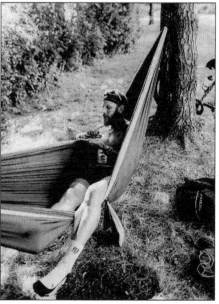

Falling asleep while being adjusted in
North Carolina.

T2 in Maine.

IRON COWBOY

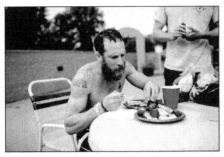

Ten thousand calories a day isn't easy.

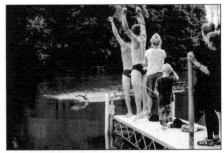

The best cheerleaders in the world.

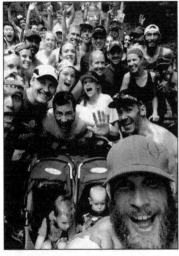

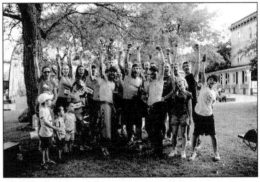

Play time in New York.

Run crowd in Massachusetts.

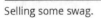

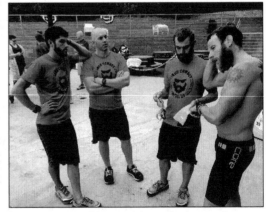

Selling some swag.

Casey, Dallas and Aaron giving a tired pep talk.

PHOTO COLLAGE

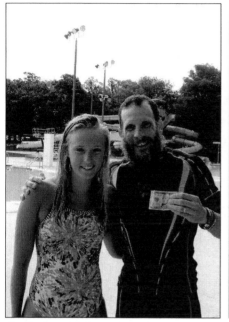
Charity found at the bottom of a pool swim.

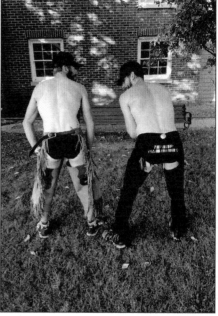
Racing in full costume in New York.

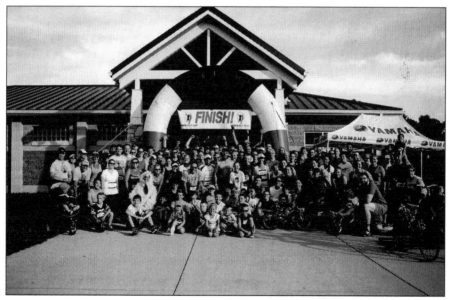
The amazing support continues in Indiana

IRON COWBOY

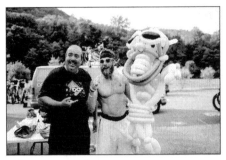

Balloon Iron Cowboy.

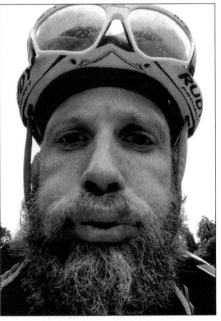

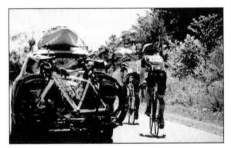

Refueling in Vermont.

Trying to stay awake on the bike.

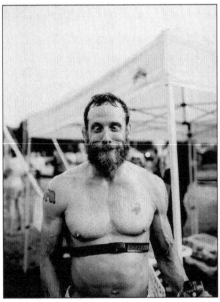

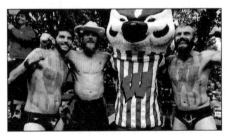

I found a new wingman in Wisconsin.

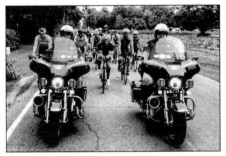

Having a little fun late in the journey.

Police Escort in Michigan.

PHOTO COLLAGE

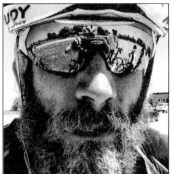

Tired in Iowa.

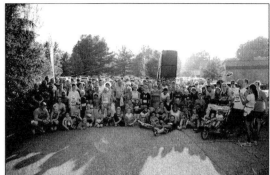

Overwhelming support in Ohio.

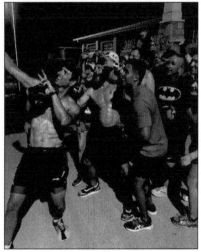

Final marathon crew in Indiana with Joe Morton.

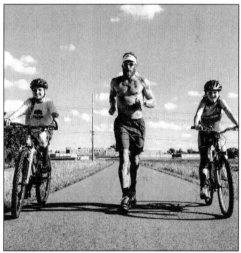

Hanging out with Lucy and Lily in South Dakota.

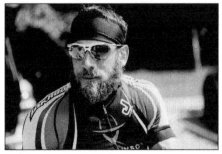

Looking for the finish.

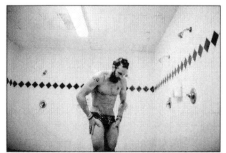

Looks like a road map on my legs.

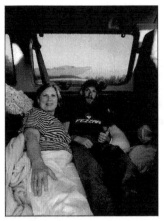

Reunited with my mother on day #45 in North Dakota.

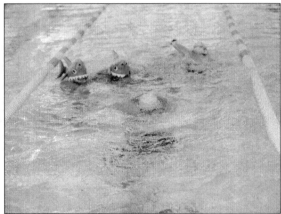

Shark attack in Idaho.

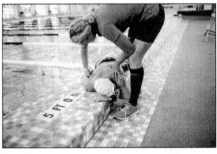

Shoulder issues.

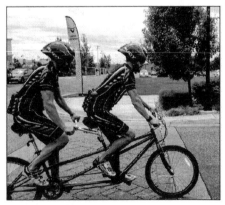

Wingmen joining me in style in Idaho.

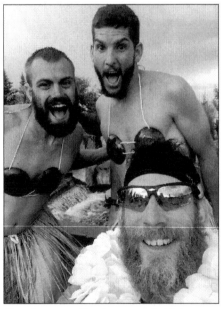

The wingmen still going strong in Idaho.

PHOTO COLLAGE

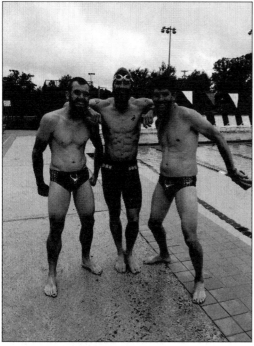

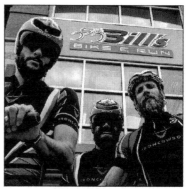

Ready to ride in Idaho.

Hanging poolside before yet another swim.

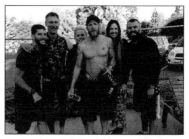

Reuniting with friends in Wyoming.

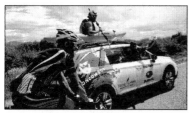

Wingmen fun in Montana.

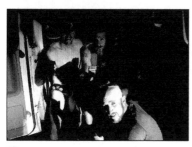

After a tough race in Wyoming.

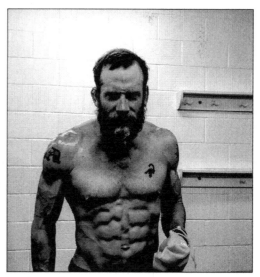

Day #48 in Wyoming, ready to be done.

IRON COWBOY

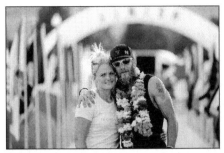

Sunny and me at the finish, reunited.

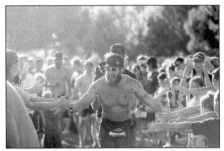

The final finish.

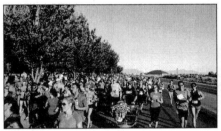

The final 5k in Utah on day #50.

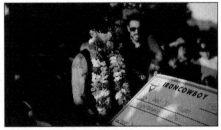

Presenting a nice big check to the Foundation.

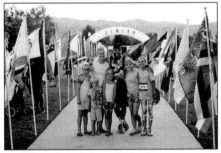

One of my favorite memories.

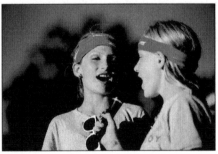

Lucy and Lily signing at the finale.

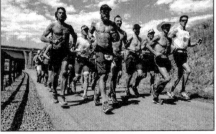

Final marathon.

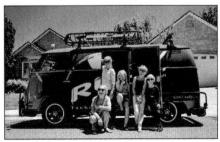

Post #50 Photo Shoot.

PHOTO COLLAGE

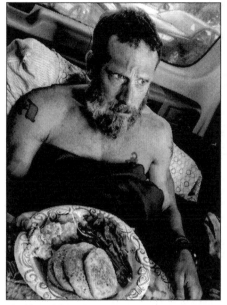

Final breakfast after a very cold swim in Utah.

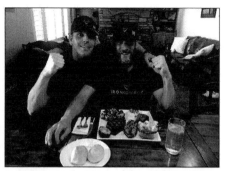

Post #50 meal with good friend Garen Winn.

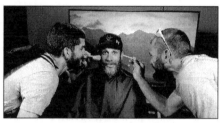

Powder prep from the wingmen.

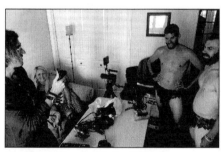

Rich Roll Podcast with the Wingmen.

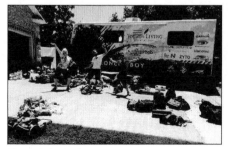

Cleanup in Utah.

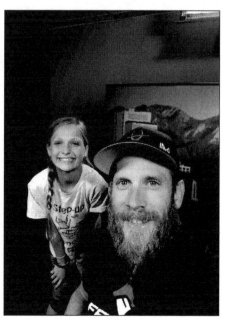

Fox News with my daughter Lucy.

THANK YOU
TO OUR SPONSORS

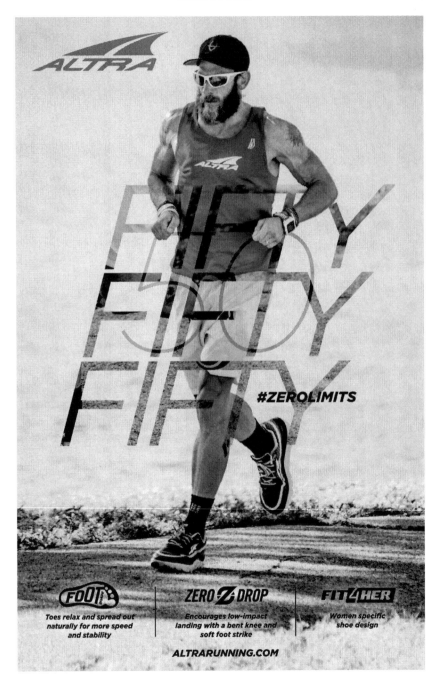

SPONSORS

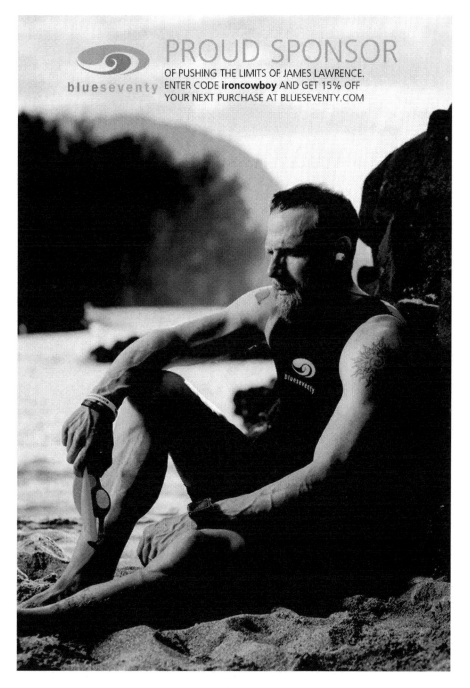

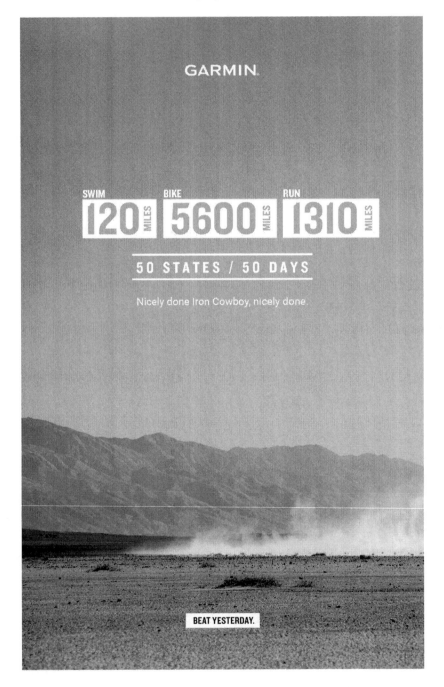

GARMIN.

SWIM | BIKE | RUN
120 MILES | 5600 MILES | 1310 MILES

50 STATES / 50 DAYS

Nicely done Iron Cowboy, nicely done.

BEAT YESTERDAY.

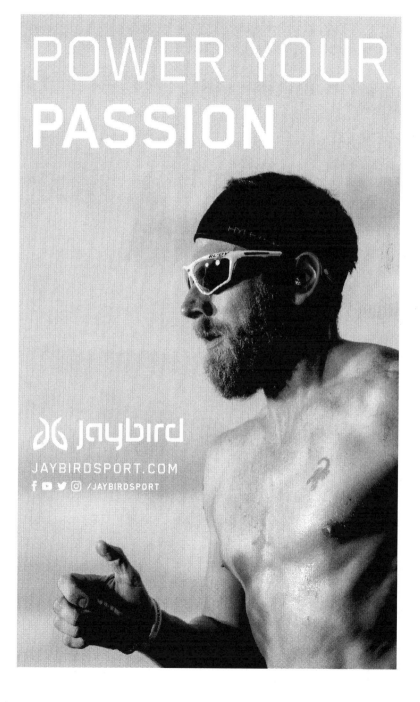

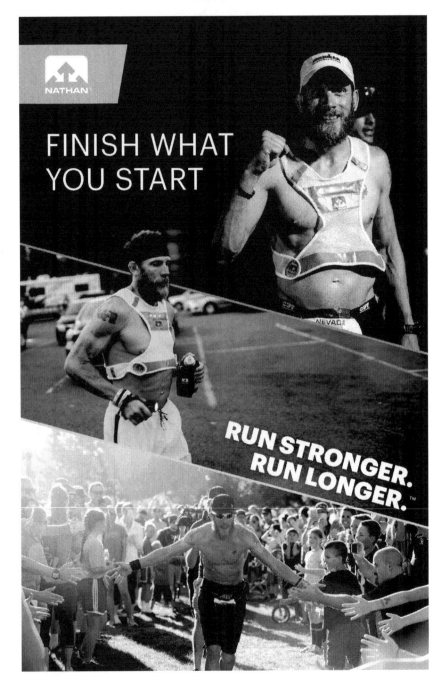

SPONSORS

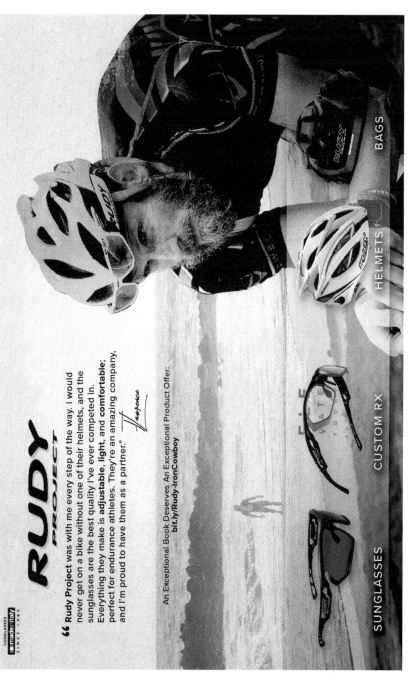

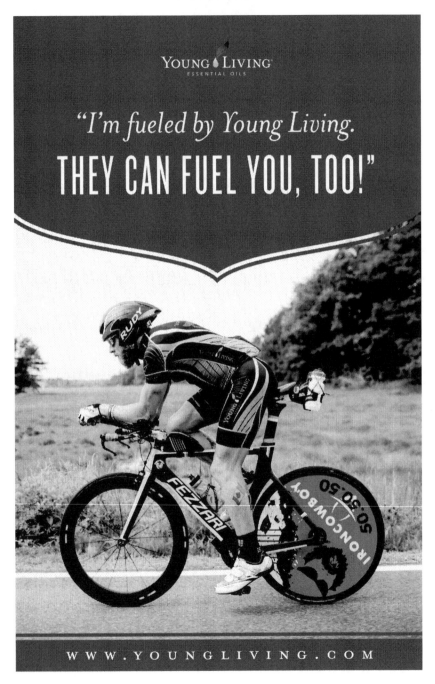

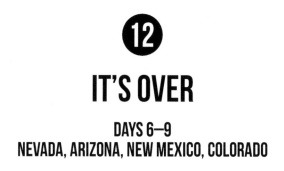

IT'S OVER

DAYS 6–9
NEVADA, ARIZONA, NEW MEXICO, COLORADO

We pulled into a mostly empty parking lot at the Heritage Park Aquatic Complex in Henderson, Nevada, at seven thirty in the morning on Day 6, after a nine-hour drive from Santa Cruz. The newly constructed building that stood before us looked like third place in a modern design contest, its façade a collision of sharp shapes and shiny materials. We crawled like rusted tin men out of the Subaru—Aaron from the driver's seat, Brittany from the front passenger seat, and I from the back—and passed through glass doors into a concourse-like interior with clean white walls and huge multi-paned windows letting in pale desert sunlight. Although the pool's fourteen lanes were nearly empty, I plunged into one that was already in use by a senior man with a full gray beard who swam with a snorkel. When he noticed me he shouted my name and hugged me like a long-lost friend.

Barry and I had, in fact, met only once before, at a conference held earlier in the year in New York City. His overflowing positivity—the way Barry treated each moment as a gift—had made a strong impression on me. From his own lips, I learned he had not always been this way. In 2004, Barry got out of bed from an afternoon nap and collapsed to the floor, suddenly unable to control his limbs. He was rushed to the hospital, where baffled doctors subjected him to a series of tests before eventually diagnosing him with Guillain-Barre Syndrome, a rare neurological disease that paralyzes its victims. Barry spent the next two-plus years bedridden, and then he passed another three years in a wheelchair before slowly regaining the ability to walk. He started swimming on the advice of a friend and found it so beneficial, both physically and mentally, that by the time I met him he was swimming three miles or more every day. Still looking for inspiration anywhere he could find it, Barry had flown to Las Vegas from his home in Los Angeles with his full-time medical assistant just to swim with me today.

Releasing me from his embrace, Barry got back to his workout, and I got started on iron-distance triathlon number six. A single stroke revealed that my injured right shoulder was not improved—indeed, it was worse than ever. After a few unpleasant laps I paused at the wall and tried to hoist myself out of the pool so that Brittany could offer my muscles some relief, but my lame arm buckled, and I splashed back in. Brittany crouched down and dragged me up onto the deck, where I lay prostrate on the clammy tiles, a position that was less conducive to treatment than it was symbolic of my psychological state.

"What do you need me to do?" Brittany asked.

"I don't know," I said. "Nothing helps."

Brittany did what she could, and I returned to the water, but the pain continued to intensify until it exceeded the limit of tolerability. Continuing to use my right arm was as impossible as keeping a bare palm in contact with a hot burner. I had no choice but to tuck my right arm against my body like a broken wing and stroke with my left arm only. This worked just as well as swimming with both arms—except it was a lot slower and took twice as much energy and made breathing awkward, causing me to swallow a lot of water.

I still had the better part of a mile left to cover when Barry, having completed his three miles and having a plane to catch, bid me farewell. Sixty-six years old and a recent quadriplegic, he too struggled to hoist himself out of the pool—but not as much as I had.

While I thrashed from wall to wall like a wounded duck, my friend Kyle arrived from Utah bearing instant oatmeal, bananas, honey, and antifungal cream and Gold Bond powder for my toe blisters. While I ate my oats, Brittany taped my shoulder and applied the cream and powder to my feet, going extra heavy on the infected right foot.

"You owe me free coaching for life for this," Brittany said.

I started my bike ride right outside the aquatic center, accompanied by Brittany, Kyle, and my friends Tim and John. Everyone had driven from Utah except Tim; he had driven up from California. It felt like a Saturday group ride back home.

The feeling didn't last. Three hours later, our shattered group was stalled at the side of

⑫ IT'S OVER

Highway 95 under a glaring sun. Tim was leaning against a traffic sign, dry heaving. John's jersey and shorts were torn open, revealing abrasions acquired in an earlier crash. Brittany had crashed as well and was now recovering in the Subaru. Kyle and I were in the process of exchanging bikes, a giant screw having shredded my front tire.

Just then, Natalie and the wingmen arrived in a rented vehicle with my cooling sleeves—a pair of sun-deflecting white sleeves that are soaked in ice water and worn on the arms—which I had requested in an earlier phone call.

"What happened?" Natalie asked, taking in the tableau of defeat.

"I'm getting all my bad luck out of the way early today," I said.

I flatted three more times in the remaining fifty miles of the bike ride.

It was almost midnight when I completed my marathon at Reunion Trails Park, a hilltop recreation area with a view of the garish lights of the Las Vegas strip some twelve miles to the north. While Sunny put the kids to bed inside the RV and the crew packed up for the long drive to Flagstaff, I talked to Ron, a writer for the *Las Vegas Review-Journal*.

"Is it true you rode a Ferris wheel for ten days?" he asked.

"Hardest thing I've ever done," I said.

I have a theory: if you can make a joke, you can take another step.

A dull impact between the motor home and something living woke me with a jolt. I called out to Casey from my bed.

"You hit something. Pull over."

"I don't think so," Casey lied.

"I think you hit a deer," I said.

He finally pulled over. Sunny, Casey and I stepped out into the brisk, early morning to inspect the damage. The whole right headlight assembly had been ripped away. Aaron, who'd been trailing us in the Subaru, approached on foot.

"You hit a deer," he said. "I saw fur everywhere."

Casey gave me a guilty look. He was well aware I had once hit a deer while driving late at night, just 30 hours before my wedding. My car went off the road, rolled four times, and was totaled, leaving us to borrow a car for our wedding. I've had a phobia of hitting deer ever since.

Sleep eluded me during the ninety minutes that remained in our journey to

IRON COWBOY

Upper Lake Mary, east of Flagstaff. Casey parked next to a gray twelve-passenger van that held eight people and a rubber raft. One of those eight people was Dayton, the boy I had pushed and pulled through Ironman Arizona in 2012. The others were his parents, Sherrine and Wes, and his five brothers and sisters. Of all the naively hopeful assumptions I had made when planning the Fifty, the naivest of all was imagining that I would be up to the task of pulling and pushing Dayton. They had driven from the Phoenix area to join me in today's triathlon.

As I squeezed my body inside my wetsuit, I explained plan B to Sherrine: Casey would tug Dayton's raft through the swim, Aaron would pull his trailer over the bike course, and we'd see about the run. Sherrine could not mask her disappointment.

I chose to enter Lake Mary via a concrete boat ramp that appeared to extend into the water but (I would soon find out) stopped abruptly right at the water line. When I stepped into the lake, my reaching foot found nothing solid to rest on, and I fell spectacularly, gashing my heel on a sharp rock.

My poor feet.

I swam again with one arm, and like the day before it was as exhausting as pedaling a bike with only one leg. Unfortunately, today I was in open water, so I couldn't pause at a wall as necessary to catch my breath. A couple of hundred yards from shore, I paused anyway, lungs heaving. The most prominent object in my field of vision was Dayton's raft.

Dayton's raft.

I flung out my left arm and grabbed hold of it. Dayton gave me a sidelong look. His expressions don't change much, but the subtlest shift in the set of his features seemed to say, *Uh-oh.* Casey, feeling the additional drag, stopped swimming and looked at me quizzically.

"I'm toast," I told him. "My shoulder's completely shot. I don't think I can make it with one arm."

"You have to keep going," Casey said.

Gee, thanks for the sympathy.

Pissed off by my wingman's tough-guy attitude, I put my head down and continued swimming.

According to scientists, anger increases pain tolerance. They're right. When I paused a second time to rest and check my watch, I was outraged to see how little progress I had made. I put my head back down and swam some more, my pain tolerance further heightened.

142

⑫ IT'S OVER

Several more cycles of angry swimming and desperate clinging to Dayton's raft brought me to the swim's midpoint. Turning around, I cursed myself for having swum straight out from shore. The boat launch looked impossibly far away. The motorhome was the size of a toy, and the people were just specks of color. My left shoulder felt rubbery with fatigue—and now my anger turned to fear.

Fifty-three minutes later, I lurched out of the lake and staggered into the gathering of family, crew, and supporters waiting for me at the water's edge. My friend Mike was there, having driven up from the Phoenix area. Mike was a friend of mine from Utah; in fact, he was my boss at the golf course I worked at when Sunny and I first got married. We became close friends quickly and spent a lot of time together. He was there to witness my first marathon, my first season of triathlon, and my first iron distance triathlon. Time had come between us, but when I saw his smile, it felt like old times.

I did not immediately notice the presence of my friend Rivers, an elite ultra-runner who lived in Flagstaff and had just arrived on his mountain bike. When he stepped forward to say hello, I saw that his eyes were red-rimmed. Only later would I learn, secondhand, that Rivers had seen me swimming from a distance as he pedaled his way toward the lake. Before that moment, he'd been certain I would fail to achieve my goal. Having been moved to tears by the sight of me swimming with one arm, he now believed nothing could stop me.

I put Rivers right to work peeling my wetsuit off. With teeth chattering (the air temperature was forty-one degrees), I slipped into the motorhome to eat and change. When I came back out, Dayton's trailer was hooked up to Aaron's bike, and Sherrine and Rivers were also ready to ride.

We rolled along Lake Mary Road, toward Mormon Lake. Five miles in, we started to climb. I kept an eye on my power meter, respecting the 140-watt limit David had told me not to exceed lest I burn myself out, but the effort felt much harder than normal. Then I remembered I was at 7,000 feet.

"Remind me why I picked Flagstaff," I grumbled.

Aaron couldn't keep up. By the time Rivers and I had summited the climb, he, Dayton, and Sherrine were out of sight behind us. We would not see them again. At thirty-two miles, we hit the second climb, this one even more formidable, ascending 600 feet over four miles.

We were supposed to circle Mormon Lake twice, but after the first circuit, I begged Rivers to take me someplace flatter. "I don't care if I have to circle a parking lot," I said.

Eventually, we found a relatively flat five-mile stretch of road between the boat launch and the Lake Mary Country Store, a quaint little shop where Rivers was very pleased to score twenty Red Vines for a dollar. Back and forth we went, picking up one or two new supporters each time we returned to the staging area.

By this point, my feet were killing me. They had swollen so much over the past several days that my toenails scraped against the tops of my cycling shoes at the apex of each pedal stroke, creating new blisters and exacerbating existing ones. Rivers suggested I ride with my feet on top of the shoes. This brought some relief, but at the cost of greatly reducing my pedaling efficiency.

Our planned stopping point was a Whole Foods store in Flagstaff where we had invited people who were interested in running with me to meet up. Rivers had miscalculated the distance, and when we hit 112 miles, we were still three miles away. I stopped cold and pulled out my phone to call the wingmen and request a pickup. No signal. With a disgusted shake of the head, I put my feet back on top of my shoes and slow-pedaled in a low gear to the staging area.

I figured Rivers owed me one for causing me to ride the extra distance, so I asked him for a massage. He wasn't a massage therapist, but he was enrolled in physical therapy school and had learned the basics of the art. As Casey and Aaron looked on, I lay down on a foldout massage table inside the motor home and Rivers removed his sweaty jersey, dropped the straps of his bib shorts, and oiled up his hands and forearms.

"Wait, I thought the person *getting* the massage was supposed to get naked, not the one giving it," Aaron said.

We all cackled like lunatics.

Five hours later, nothing was funny. I was walking along Lake Mary Road toward Flagstaff in total darkness, or what would have been total darkness if not for the light shed by two vehicles, a van creeping ahead of the Subaru and me, driven by Sunny, trailing behind. I had seven miles left in my marathon, and I could not feel my legs below the knees. A pair of knee braces I had put on earlier after feeling a twinge on the right side was causing fluid to pool in my lower legs. The obvious solution was to remove them, but I was so brainless from exhaustion and dehydration that I had not made the connection, so the braces stayed on, and the condition worsened.

I had plenty of company, at least. Lucy, Lily, the wingmen, Sherrine, Dayton,

⓵⓶ IT'S OVER

a guy from Mesa who was pushing Dayton, an eleven-year-old boy named Walter, whom my girls had befriended, and several local supporters were cocooning me, urging me on, giving me food and drink. When I complained of a rock in my shoe, a stranger knelt down and extracted it while a couple of others held me up.

I kept telling myself to take just one more step. But each step sapped a little more of my dwindling willpower. There came a moment between steps when I tried to reach inside myself for another fistful of resolve, and I came up empty. For the first time in my life, I could not muster the motivation to take one more step.

Suddenly, as if controlled by an invisible puppeteer, I veered off the road and plopped down on a patch of grass, where I curled into a ball with my forehead pressed against my knees. Lucy rushed over to me, grabbed one of my hands in both of hers, and tried to yank me upright.

"Come on, Dad!" she said. "You have to finish!"

I got back up and resumed hobbling, using my daughter's determination as a substitute for my own.

"How much farther?" I mumbled.

"A little more than five miles," Casey said.

Five miles! It was unimaginable. In utter despair, I sat down a second time. Lucy again tried to goad me back into action.

"I think he really needs to sit," protested one of the local women in our group.

"I think he needs to get up!" Lucy shot back.

I stood up in a tottering sort of way, like a bruised and bloodied boxer dragging himself off the canvas for the final knockout. I took one step, then another. Each step was preceded by an argument between two distinct inner voices, like this:

I can't.

Do it anyway.

Step.

I can't.

Do it anyway.

Step.

We crept slowly into civilization, the density of lights, stores, restaurants, and vehicular traffic gradually increasing. Aaron spied a Five Guys and sprinted toward it.

"I need a cup of pickle juice," he blurted at a bemused cashier.

Pickle juice is believed to alleviate muscle cramps. What I had was something close to the *opposite* of muscle cramps, but when Aaron handed me the cup, I drank it automatically.

We made a right turn onto Butler Avenue. Suddenly, college students were all around us. It was a Friday night in a university town, and everyone was hell-bent on fun. Another twenty minutes of walking brought us back to the parking lot of Whole Foods, where a few people who had been promised the opportunity to run with me at seven would instead get to walk with me at eleven.

Halfway through an Iron Cowboy 5K that looked and felt more like a funeral procession, I asked Aaron to hurry back to the motorhome and fetch Dallas, who had just flown in from Utah. When Aaron returned with Dallas, I told my chiropractor about my dead legs. He knelt and pulled the knee braces down around my ankles. Instantly I felt the tiniest bit of relief—not enough to save me from my plight, but more than enough to teach me I had brought the crisis on myself.

Completing the 5K left me with about two miles to cover. I was now unable to step up onto or down from curbs without assistance, so Casey and Aaron decided I would finish up my seven-and-a-half-hour marathon by pacing back and forth across the parking lot within sight of the motor home.

As I shuffled along, I discovered that I felt ever so slightly, less miserable, if I closed my eyes. Moments later, I was startled back to consciousness by strong hands gripping my upper arms. The wingmen had seen me teeter and caught me just in time. They kept hold of me and frog-marched me to the next turnaround point, where Aaron lifted my arm to squint at my watch and see how far I had to go, and then Casey rotated me 180 degrees for the next segment.

At last, the ordeal ended. It was time to thank my few remaining supporters and have photos taken with them. Instead, I just stood outside the motorhome with my head down. Casey cleared his throat and spoke on my behalf. "I'm sorry it was such a rough day," he said, voice quavering. "Thank you for believing in James. Because we do."

I turned my back to the group and reeled toward the door of the motorhome, forgetting to say good-bye even to Dayton, who'd been let down more than anyone on this miserable day. Seeing that the steps presented an insurmountable obstacle, Casey and Aaron shoved me inside like a shackled prisoner.

Sunny was there waiting for me. She looked at me with hope, yet empathy. I gazed at her in silence. Each of us was waiting for the other to speak.

"It's over," I finally said.

⑫ IT'S OVER

Kyle's head appeared in the window of the Toyota Tundra Double Cab, in whose backseat I lay drifting in and out of sleep. The truck was parked on the shoulder of Highway 50, the only silver dot glinting on a vast, empty high-desert moonscape north of Albuquerque, New Mexico.

"You look terrible," Kyle said.

I did look terrible; my skin had acquired a deathly gray pallor, there was a far-away look in my eyes, and I had lost seven pounds since the start of the campaign. My gaunt face looked ten years older than it had eight days before. I said nothing.

"I found the bike shoes," Kyle said in a different tone, showing me a glossy new pair of white Shimano TR32s. More important than the color or the brand was the size: thirteen, to accommodate my swollen, infected, blistered size twelve feet.

I mumbled my thanks and sank back into sleep. Kyle shook me awake.

"We have an IV set up for you too," he said. "A nurse is going to meet us at the motorhome. Do you think you can ride there?"

I said I thought I could, then fell asleep again. Kyle shook me awake once more and helped me out of the backseat.

The day had started well—miraculously well, in fact. When I was woken up inside the motorhome upon arriving in Albuquerque, my NormaTec compression boots were still running. On the drive from Flagstaff, Dallas had thrown every trick he knew at my monstrously swollen and almost untouchable painful lower legs—acupuncture, active release therapy, a cold laser treatment—before strapping the boots on as I slept. I removed them and saw that the swelling was gone. I touched the skin and felt no pain.

My luck ended there. No matter his skill and talent, Dallas was unable to work similar magic on my ailing right shoulder, and I was forced to swim all but the first nine laps of my outdoor pool swim at Riverpoint Sports and Wellness with one arm. After the third pause for treatment had resulted in zero improvements, discouragement pressed down on me like an external weight. I thought about not just the two-plus miles I had to swim this morning, but also the forty-one swims I would have to complete in the next six weeks. In all likelihood, my shoulder would become even more painful and useless as the campaign wore on unless I continued not to use it. And how much one-armed swimming could I do before my overburdened left shoulder blew out?

Reading my thoughts, Sunny leaped into the pool and began to tread water in the lane next to mine, speaking each time I passed.

"Forget about tomorrow," she said. "Forget about the next lap. Take it one stroke at a time, baby."

Sunny's recitation of my own philosophy did not soothe my pain nor lessen my discouragement, but it made me feel less alone in my pain and discouragement, and that was something.

My friends Ron and Cathy had come from Utah and were poolside, encouraging me as I swam. Heath Haacke also came from Utah and planned to do the whole day with me. He swam in his own lane, to stay out of my way, and continued his swim as I indulged in two pans of food: eggs and hash browns. I sat in the hot tub enjoying the hot water and my favorite breakfast foods.

On the bike, I traded shoulder pain for tunnel vision and blackouts, which started about an hour after I'd set out from the club with a few supporters. By the time I hit the third or fourth instance of snapping awake, on the brink of tipping over, it scared me enough that I pulled my phone out of my pocket and made a call. My New Mexico ambassador, Gene, who'd been trailing me in his truck with his wife, Joan, answered and I asked him to stop so I could catch a few winks.

I dismounted and handed my bike to my friend Heath, with my shoes still clipped to the pedals (as in Flagstaff, I'd been riding with my feet on top of them). My first step toward the truck brought my right heel down on a pile of goat head thorns, nature's thumbtacks. I opened my mouth in a silent scream, lifted the insulted foot off the ground, lost my balance, and fell into Gene's arms. He and Heath stuffed me into the truck, where Kyle woke me more than an hour later.

The motorhome was parked seventeen miles away at the Alameda Open Space in North Albuquerque. My supporters formed a protective pod around me and kept me alert by chattering away and asking questions as we rode, but my attention was on the western sky, where I saw gunmetal-gray thunderclouds rolling toward us. The winds picked up, and the temperature plunged.

I had just reached the safety of the motorhome when the sky cracked open. The nurse Kyle had spoken of was waiting for me inside. She slipped the needle in and left me to rest on one of the twin beds in back, where the kids slept at night. Twenty minutes later, I woke up on my own, just as the rain was letting up and the last drops of saline were emptying from the bag, which Kyle had hung from a bike rack on the back of the RV, the tube snaked through an open window. I felt like a new man.

When Kyle came back to check on me, he found me rummaging in a cooler for a drink and a snack. He froze, looking at me as though I had just risen from the dead. "Let's go," I said.

When I stepped outside to face the last sixty miles of my bike ride, I was amazed to find that my riding companions were still there waiting for me. One of these hardy loyalists, Ira, had run and walked with me the night before in Flagstaff. Stirred by my struggle, he had made a spur-of-the-moment decision to cannonball through the night to Albuquerque, where he borrowed a bike and bought compression underwear from Walmart to ride in. Another guy, Steve, had never ridden farther than one hundred miles on his bike, but elected to complete the full 112 with me after seeing my condition.

Later, during the Iron Cowboy 5K, I met three young children whose parents had dropped everything and rushed there from Utah after reading about my rough day in Flagstaff on Facebook. I could scarcely process what was happening. Some kind of sympathetic grassroots rescue operation had spontaneously coalesced around me, all of these strangers motivated independently of one another to help me, at great inconvenience to themselves, in the only way they could: by showing up. Even Kyle's two sons got caught up in the movement, running six miles with me. As young as they were, they too responded to the intensity of my passion and were touched by the depths of suffering I was willing to endure to fulfill my dream, which, for one enchanted hour on a warm night in Albuquerque, became their dream too.

Day 9 started with a tense exchange between my Colorado ambassador, Eric, and my crew outside the Colorado State University Student Recreation Center in Pueblo. We were supposed to have shown up at six o'clock. Not only did we roll in ninety minutes late, but nobody from our party had bothered to contact Eric and notify him, leaving him to plead with the facility manager who had opened the pool just for us (it was Sunday) not to lock up and leave. When at last we did arrive, Eric made sure we appreciated the awkwardness of the position we'd put him in.

The facility manager did all but tap his watch to demonstrate his impatience for our departure, but I refused to be rushed. My priority was food. Kyle asked Matthew, a local runner who had come out to provide SAG support during my bike ride, if the facility had a microwave he could use to heat up some instant oatmeal. Matthew zipped home and returned with oatmeal from his house. Stomach appeased, I got in the pool.

Casey swam ahead of me, creating a slipstream I was able to glide in with about 15 percent less effort—and 15 percent less strain on my ruined right shoulder—than if I had been alone. After a wardrobe change and a second breakfast (scrambled eggs, hash browns, and toast that Kyle brought from a nearby Denny's), I mounted my bike. The only person to start with me was my friend and former coach Sonja, who had driven down from Denver. I was happy to see her, but too tired to show it. Her own warm smile of recognition turned into a frown of concern when I greeted her in a raspy whisper outside the recreation center.

We started out heading east on Highway 47 toward the airport. It was a fine morning: sixty degrees, clear-skied, the air thin and fresh.

"So how *are* you?" Sonja asked.

Her emphasis on the third word gave the question a whole different meaning.

"You can't imagine what I'm going through," I said.

"How are you dealing with it?" she asked.

I thought about this for a minute. "I wouldn't ever say this publicly," I said, "but I get a lot of strength from thinking about prisoners of war. As much as I'm suffering, it's nothing compared to being tortured and starved and locked up 10,000 miles from home. Plus, I'm doing this by choice; I have control. It's only fifty days. I think about how they fought to survive, and fighting was the only choice they had."

The weather turned. At sixty miles, a lashing rain began to fall, driven sideways by a fierce northwest wind. When the rain became hail, Matthew, who'd been following us all morning and into the afternoon in his SUV, pulled off the road and we scrambled inside. Shivering violently, I noticed an empty granola bar wrapper on the floor between my feet. I picked it up and showed it to Matthew.

"Got any more of these?" I asked.

There were two more. Matthew had been counting on their calories to get him through the rest of his long day of support work. Instead, he respectfully handed them over, and I ate them.

Four hours later, a pack of twenty-nine runners led by a bearded dreamer set out from Vitamin Cottage Natural Grocers and rambled south toward the Pueblo Riverwalk, spilling onto the streets and mildly annoying motorists. We squeezed eight miles in before seven o'clock p.m. Among the additional runners who joined us then

⑫ IT'S OVER

for the Iron Cowboy 5K were Lucy, Lily, and Daisy, who cheerfully recounted their day at an Airbnb house as we clicked off eleven-minute miles.

"We found a big frog in the backyard!" Daisy announced.

"Did you make frog soup with him?" I teased.

All three girls squealed and protested.

"No, we were nice to him!" Lily said.

"We built him a castle!" Dolly added.

"We got to ride a horse," Lily and Daisy said in unison.

"The house smelled old," Quinn said, as he stuck his tongue out.

Sunny and the kids left in the motorhome immediately after the 5K to get a head start on the 432-mile drive to Wichita. Jordan and Jessa stayed behind with the van, which had been partially emptied to make room for a more comfortable sleeping pallet than the one I'd tossed and turned on in the Subaru the night before.

Our diminished group continued on a 1.1-mile loop around the river walk that was bathed in the soft light of old-fashioned street lamps. Someone handed me a bag full of Taco Bell, and I snarfed its contents with doglike greed. I had never eaten so much fast food.

At eighteen miles, I felt an alarming twinge in my right thigh. Instantly my attention became wholly absorbed in the silver-dollar-size knot of pain emanating from deep inside my quadriceps. I prayed it was just a cramp that would work itself out if I kept going, but the longer the feeling persisted, the more confident I became that I had strained a muscle. I was forced to transition from a limping run to a herky-jerky power walk. Sonja, still with me, asked what was wrong, and I told her. Her expression turned grave. She was an experienced enough athlete herself to know that an acute muscle strain might be fatal to my ambitions.

Sunny and I believe most injuries have an emotional component. I texted Sunny, asking her to help me identify the source of this latest bodily mutiny. She consulted her copy of *Messages from the Body* and texted me back: "Worrying too much about details. Trying to control everything."

My skin went tingly with recognition. It was true. I had been wasting a lot of energy fretting about aspects of the campaign other than swimming, cycling, and running. Could I just snap my fingers and give up control, click my heels together and stop worrying? Our operation so far had been chaotic and dysfunctional. The motorhome looked as if burglars had ransacked it. Sponsors and supporters were riding us for slacking on the social media front. Online haters and trolls were accusing me of charity fraud because things still weren't properly lined up with the Jamie Oliver Food Foundation. In Flagstaff, I'd laid into Casey and Aaron when I'd found them goofing around at the staging area when one of them could have been catching up on badly needed sleep while the other attended to me. And this afternoon, Eric had called Aaron and asked him what had happened to the guy (Jordan) who was supposed to be supporting me while I rode. Answer: he'd gone off to have a picnic with his wife and her family.

These things were well worth worrying about, but I knew I needed to let them go. If I persisted in trying to carry everything on my shoulders, my body would disintegrate, muscle by muscle, bone by bone, joint by joint.

I began to speak healing statements. "I forgive myself for believing my team isn't handling their tasks," I said. "I forgive myself for believing that I need to control everything."

Sonja echoed each of these affirmations. As the process continued, a plump tear gathered at the base of my eye, broke loose, and rolled down my cheek. Then came another. When the waterworks stopped, I felt better. I began to look on the bright side of my situation. Things *were* improving. Before returning home to Utah with his sons, Kyle had instituted new routines and procedures, including a bin system for separating and organizing my swim, bike, and run gear. Sunny, Jordan, and Jessa had spent much of the evening restoring order to the items in the van and motorhome. During the previous day's marathon, we'd done our first live Periscope broadcast, and our social media following had eaten it up.

I continued to power walk. A few of my ten remaining companions had to jog to keep pace with my quick shuffle. Time was a concern. I had planned to take an IV from Eric (who, conveniently, worked as a nurse and paramedic) after completing the marathon, but I now doubted I could afford the twenty minutes. Suddenly an idea came to me.

"Can I walk with an IV?" I asked Eric, who was jogging beside me in pink flip-flops.

"I don't see why not," he said.

The next time we swung by the staging area, Eric grabbed a saline bag. Hooking it up was a cinch because he'd left a catheter in my arm after administering an earlier drip. Eric held the bag aloft as I speed-walked the last three miles, my surviving companions merrily snapping photos of the ghoulish spectacle.

When I was done, I thanked and hugged everyone and grinned for more pho-

⑫ IT'S OVER

tos. As people began to disperse, I caught sight of Matthew, walking away in the distance with his head down. He had never heard of me until forty-eight hours before, when he saw something about me on Facebook, and yet he had sacrificed himself for me today like the most loyal Iron Cowboy follower.

"Hey, Matthew!" I called. "Come back here!"

He came back.

"You were my guardian angel today," I told him. "I appreciate it."

Shy and quiet, Matthew had volunteered little information about himself over the course of the day, but I now got him to open up a bit. I learned that he worked as a correctional officer and that he'd started running fairly recently after being diagnosed with type 2 diabetes. He had already lost forty-five pounds.

We took a couple of selfies and said a proper good-bye. Then I crawled into the back of the van for the long drive to Kansas. As I drifted off to sleep, I wondered how many more Matthews were out there, counting on me not to fail, for reasons I might never know.

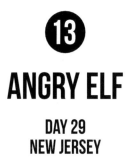

ANGRY ELF

DAY 29
NEW JERSEY

It wasn't the Iron Cowboy or even James Lawrence who slunk out of the motorhome in front of the BeachWalk at Sea Bright, our New Jersey headquarters, on the morning of Day 29, but Angry Elf. Our family loves to use the term Angry Elf when someone is in a bad mood, to use humor in acknowledging a sour mood. We borrowed it from a line in our favorite Will Ferrell movie, Elf. I was the world-hating version of me when I showed up that morning, sleep-deprived, stressed out and feeling sorry for myself. I'd been waking up as Angry Elf almost every morning lately, but on this particular morning, for whatever reason, it seemed I hated the world with increased vehemence.

Two unsuspecting welcomers immediately stepped forward to introduce themselves: Charlie, a local councilman, and Peter, whom I'd gotten to know a few years before through a former sponsor.

"Welcome to New Jersey!" Charlie boomed.

"I'm grumpy in the morning," I mumbled back.

Unfazed, Charlie explained to me there was no great rush to head over to the swim start—which lay about three miles north—because the tide had not yet turned in the Shrewsbury River. I didn't know exactly what this meant except that I didn't have to swim yet. Without speaking another word, I made a beeline for the Subaru, where I could wait in peace and quiet without having to pretend to be friendly to anyone.

I sat in the front passenger seat, semi-reclined, head lolling against the headrest, staring at nothing. Casey and Aaron, feeling equally obligated to keep me company and not to leave our hosts hanging, shuttled back and forth between us. When they were with me, the wingmen said little, knowing very well they were dealing with Angry Elf. After fifteen or twenty minutes, Charlie came to the window and said we could leave whenever I was ready. I was not ready. The prospect of another cold, shoulder-killing 2.4-mile swim made me want to set something on fire. As I continued to fume silently, I found myself unfairly blaming New Jersey for my current funk and expecting nothing but trouble from the state. At last, I gave a slight nod of the head, and Aaron turned the key in the ignition.

Sea Bright is a tiny town of 700 souls that sits on a razor-thin peninsula at the Jersey Shore, a pinky finger of eroding sand pinched between the rising Atlantic Ocean on one side and the salt water Shrewsbury River on the other. We crept along Ocean Avenue, the town's only road until we reached the entrance to Gateway National Recreation Area, known to locals as Sandy Hook, where a ranger waved us through and directed us to Lot C. More than twenty other vehicles were already present, their recent occupants huddled on the beach, waiting for me. I braced myself.

The moment I emerged from the car, I was swarmed with support. A local chiropractor, Kosta, told me he would be at my service all day. A reporter for redbankgreen.com, a local cultural website, pulled me aside for a short interview. An older fellow named Ken told me he would serve as my swim guide. He then launched into a detailed description of the swim course, but I cut him off. "I'll just follow you," I said.

A group photo was taken, and then we trooped into the river, where two paddleboarders and a pontoon boat (piloted by Charlie) waited to escort us back to Sea Bright. As I stood facing downriver in waist-deep water, I realized why Charlie had wanted me to wait for the tide to turn. A powerful current pressed against my backside with the force of a Jacuzzi jet. When I plunged in and began to stroke, a kind of liquid gravity drove me ahead like a bodysurfer. Almost despite myself, I felt my mood turning.

About half a mile into the free ride, we passed under the Highlands-Sea Bright Bridge, which connects the peninsula to the New Jersey mainland. I flipped over onto my back and shouted, my joyful voice echoing off the roadway above. "New Jersey! Best swim ever!" Seconds later, my right hamstring cramped viciously. I stopped stroking and straightened my leg to stretch out and relax the seizing muscle.

⓭ ANGRY ELF

After a few minutes, the tension had dissipated enough to permit a cautious return to swimming. When I hit 2.4 miles, I stopped again and waved Charlie over for a pickup, like a fallen water-skier. When the boat drew close, I reached out for the ladder and cramped again, this time in both legs. I locked out my knees and trod water with my arms only.

"You're going to have to pull me in," I told Charlie.

Ken climbed onto the boat to assist in the operation. Grunting and huffing, the two men leaned over the stern and yanked me out of the drink, my legs as rigid as planks. From the shore, it must have appeared that a fresh corpse, stiff with rigor mortis, had been recovered. Somewhere amid the awkward fumbling with my body, a sharp pain pierced the right side of my rib cage. I had dislocated ribs before, and I was pretty sure I'd just done it again.

Ken and Charlie laid me down on the deck and piled blankets and towels on me. I closed my eyes and tried to escape to someplace far away in my mind. The double whammy of pains I'd just experienced had struck at the worst possible time, right when I had stopped bracing for the worst and had made myself vulnerable to hope. By the time Charlie's boat bumped against the pier at Sea Bright and woke me, Angry Elf was back.

My rescuers helped me up and handed me over to the wingmen on the dock. I moved like a hypothermic survivor of a cold-water capsizing. Kosta, the chiropractor, was also there to receive me. Before the swim, I'd told him that I was going to need him afterward, but I'd had no idea just how badly.

Within a few minutes, I was face down on a treatment table inside a double-queen room at the BeachWalk, plucking grapes, bananas, and halved avocados out of baskets the wingmen had conveniently placed on the floor beneath me. Kosta took my top half while another chiropractor, Jennifer, handled my legs.

As she rubbed essential oils into my calves, Jennifer spoke up hesitantly. "Your body seems to be telling me there might be an emotional source to your cramping," she said.

Kosta shot a startled glance at the wingmen.

"That wouldn't surprise me," I said.

"Are you open to exploring it?" Jennifer asked, sounding less tentative.

"Sure, why not?" I said.

Jennifer instructed me to extend my left arm (I couldn't lift the right), make a fist, and resist the downward pressure she applied to my hand with hers. I knew the drill, having done muscle testing, a widely practiced technique in alternative medi-cine, for twenty years, first with my mother and more recently with Sunny. Jennifer then named a series of negative emotions—sadness, fear, and so forth—and pressed down on my fist with each utterance. Again and again, my arm dropped with lit-tle resistance—until she mentioned *frustration*. At that point, Jennifer stopped and asked me to focus on this feeling.

"Now we're going to find the cause of your frustration," she said.

I almost laughed. *Let's see . . .could it be the endless succession of injuries? The mind-numbing tedium of exercising all day, every day? The constant exhaustion? The soul-starving scarcity of quality time with Sunny and the kids? The Internet sniping? Jordan's growing estrangement from the rest of us? The continuing sponsor headaches?*

But it wasn't until Jennifer mentioned "my team" that my arm dropped a second time. My team? This struck me as the least of my present frustrations, and yet it was weirdly consistent with Sunny's diagnosis of the source of my thigh muscle strain back in Colorado.

"Can you put *frustration* and *my team* together in a sentence for me?" Jennifer asked.

Now it was the wingmen's turn to look uncomfortable.

"I'm frustrated by the challenge of communicating my needs to my team and by the difficulty of keeping us all on the same page," I said dutifully.

Jennifer explained that frustration tends to be associated with obstruction of the liver meridian, which is located at the bottom of the right side of the rib cage— the exact location of the pain that had struck me when Charlie and Ken yanked me out of the river. She asked me to lay my left hand on that spot and the right on my forehead and to breathe deeply while meditating on my frustration with my crew. Meanwhile, Jennifer used her thumbs to apply acupressure to various points on my spine. Kosta looked like he wanted to be somewhere else. When the treatment was completed, my rib actually felt a lot better, and although I didn't know it yet, the problem would not return.

I dressed in my black Iron Cowboy cycling kit and stepped outside, where twen-ty-three people were waiting for me with their bikes. We lined up for another group photo and rolled out. Putting the full weight of my butt on the seat felt like sitting down on a mound of jacks. The nether parts of my physical person had been on a degenerative course throughout the Fifty and had now reached a point of crisis. Too much time on a bike seat had turned my groin, rectum, and the space between them into an anatomical war zone, a dumpster fire of overlapping maladies.

Problem number one was a nasty pair of internal hemorrhoids, which hurts like Hades, but were also causing me to produce alarming bloody stools. The second issue was good old-fashioned saddle soreness, unavoidable for someone who has spent more than six hours a day on a bike seat for four straight weeks. Problem number three—newer and more rapidly worsening than the first two—was severe inflammation in the veins running along my inner thighs, caused by friction between these tender areas and the bike seat.

Crossing over the Highlands-Sea Bright Bridge and pedaling west toward the posh town of Rumson, I waited for my saddle region to numb up a bit, as it always did, but today it didn't. Compounding my misery were the roads, which I discovered to be in an almost third-world state of disrepair. Rutted, bumpy, and infested with potholes, they subjected my private zone to a continuous low-grade agitation as I rattled over them. To spare myself the worst of this unpleasantness, I pedaled from a standing position as much as possible, trading pain in my nether parts for strain in my overworked quadriceps muscles. Nearly all the photos taken of me on my bike on that day show me in this posture, with a world-hating scowl on my face.

As we continued west through Red Bank (a hipster town packed with trendy watering holes, farm-to-fork restaurants, coffee shops not called Starbucks, and size-eight-and-below boutiques) and into greener Holmdel, where every third adult works for Bell Labs, my thoughts turned again to my late friend Tim. The painful knot on the back of my left knee that had caused me to fear death by a blood clot in South Carolina had gotten a lot better, but the hideous engorgement of the veins in my inner thighs was now even more worrisome. I pictured a deep red clog damming up the flow of blood, breaking loose, and moving like a pomegranate seed through a silly straw to my brain . . . My suddenly lifeless body dropping to the road . . . My children growing up fatherless.

A local triathlon coach named Brian was providing SAG support in his Jeep, driving just ahead of us and stopping periodically to supply refreshments. At the first stop, he asked me ("just out of curiosity") what kinds of physical ailments I was suffering from that people typically do not experience during a single Ironman triathlon. I took the bait and told him about my blazing behind and fiery groin, to which I had just finished applying generous quantities of Aquaphor. Brian mentioned that there happened to be an excellent orthopedist, Gerry, riding in our group, and urged me to talk to him about the situation.

IRON COWBOY

As we pressed deeper into Monmouth County, past gated mansions, horse ranches, and blueberry fields, I enacted Brian's advice. Gerry assured me that my symptoms were those typically associated with simple inflammation, not a blood clot. But he was kind enough not to dismiss my worries, instead suggesting I get a second opinion from a specialist.

"What kind of specialist?" I asked.

"Oh, maybe a vascular surgeon," he said.

The next time Brian's Jeep drew alongside us, I asked him if he could find me a vascular surgeon to with whom I could talk. He looked at me as though I had just asked him to find a leprechaun riding a unicorn. Only then did I recall that it was the Fourth of July.

"I'll see what I can do," he offered.

The farther west we went, the further back in time we seemed to go. The quaint little villages we passed through reminded me of Norman Rockwell paintings, frozen in America's postwar glory days. Man, Sunny would have loved these neighborhoods! We were approaching an intersection at the center of one of these towns when a traffic officer showed us his palm, bringing our peloton to a halt. A fire engine then crossed in front of us at 2.5 miles per hour, followed by a Boy Scout troop, an Elks Club legation, a high school marching band, a classic-car lineup—an entire Independence Day parade. I stood shaking my head at the procession as though it were a personal affront, unable to see the humor at the moment, as my companions evidently did.

About eighty miles in, approaching Englishtown, we stopped at a general store to grab drinks and snacks and to empty our bladders. A long line had formed outside the bathroom, so I waited in the parking lot with Brian and Tara, a top local triathlete in her sixties. While we chatted, a stream of pale yellow liquid began to run down Tara's legs.

"Are you peeing?" Brian asked.

"Why not?" she answered.

"You're a freaking bad-A!" Brian said.

These are my people, I thought.

We got back to Sea Bright at 3:40. I should have thanked my cycling companions and left it at that, but Angry Elf couldn't resist expressing his opinion that New Jersey had the worst roads in America. I then retreated to my hotel room and collapsed onto the treatment table, where I promptly passed out while Kosta gave me a

⓭ ANGRY ELF

second adjustment. When I woke up, Kosta called a doctor friend of his, Tom, who had agreed to talk to me about my swollen veins.

I described my symptoms and mentioned my terror of blood clots. Like Gerry, the orthopedist I'd spoken to earlier, Tom voiced complete confidence that I was in no danger of being killed by a brain embolism. He advised me to ice the inflamed area regularly and stay off my bike until the symptoms subsided.

"That's great advice, Doc," I said. "I won't ride my bike for a few days."

"Just take a little time off, and you'll recover," Tom reiterated.

"I sure will," I said. "That's really helpful. I'm so glad we talked."

The moment I hung up, Casey and Aaron, who had been biting their fists as they listened in, burst out in hysterics. To be fair, Kosta hadn't had time to fully explain to Tom who I was and what I was doing. Then again, I'm not sure it would have made any difference.

The wingmen and I suited up in American flag running shorts and jogged a few blocks to the center of Sea Bright, where we picked up eight supporters who wanted to log a few miles with me before the Iron Cowboy 5K, and from there we headed north, back toward Sandy Hook. An old Chevy Suburban, occupied by the president of the Sandy Hookers Triathlon Club, Doug, and his buddy Dave, rode ahead of us. Kosta and an EMT named Tina followed behind on bikes.

On previous days in the campaign, switching from cycling to running had brought relief to my wounded underside. Not today. The high-tech, ultra-thin, moisture-wicking material of my patriotic shorts felt like a cheese grater against my skin. I was seized by an overwhelming urge to tear them off and run like Adam through the village. It was becoming increasingly people-packed now that the skies had cleared and the private beach clubs that dominate Sea Bright's oceanfront were open, and the time for fireworks was drawing closer.

A mile or so from our starting point, we came upon our SAG vehicle, parked in a small beach access lot. I asked Doug and Dave, somewhat desperately, if either of them had any lubricant or ointment. Dave handed me a tube of something, and I turned away from the road, squeezed a generous dollop onto my palm, and stuffed my hand down my shorts, front and back.

"Why are you doing that?" asked TJ, a wide-eyed ten-year-old boy whose twin brother, PJ, was also in our group.

I took a moment to compose my thoughts.

"My legs are sore from riding my bike all day," I said.

IRON COWBOY

Close enough.

Another mile or so down the road, I passed gas loudly. Even this basic bodily function was painful and so raw and painful was the organ it utilized. My supporters pretended they hadn't heard it. Well, except one. "What do you do when you're running and you have to poop?" TJ asked.

I took another moment to compose my thoughts. "I just wait until I get to a bathroom," I said.

Sometimes. Not always.

A little farther along, TJ asked an even trickier question.

"Which state is your favorite?"

"New Jersey," I lied without hesitation.

We continued almost to the very tip of Sandy Hook, where I paused to take a photo of the New York City skyline. The locals had promised it would appear close enough to touch from this vantage, but to Angry Elf, the iconic Gotham cityscape looked as unreachable as the sun.

We came back to the Sea Bright Municipal Beach parking lot just before seven o'clock. Independence Day appeared to have become Iron Cowboy Day in this small nook of America. Nearly fifty people cheered my arrival. Lucy and Lily were busily hawking T-shirts and distributing race numbers, while Daisy, Dolly, and Quinn raced down to the beach. Someone had even gone so far as to make a gigantic poster featuring an image of me and tied it to a metal frame on wheels—the kind used for low-budget theater backdrops. I should have appreciated all the fuss the Garden State was making over me, but Angry Elf wanted none of it. Being the center of attention in a crowd is never comfortable for an introvert. For an introvert in a foul mood, it was torture. I pushed blindly through the scrum and disappeared inside the motorhome, where I found Sunny and the wingmen together. Their smiles tainted my already dark temper with a shade of jealousy. I had been in so much pain for so long that I felt indiscriminately hostile, like a Rottweiler with a tooth infection.

"I'm not doing my speech today," I pouted. "Casey, you do it."

Sunny fixed me with one of her looks. "James," she admonished, "those people out there are here to support YOU. Some of them even came from other states to see you. You're doing the speech."

I did the speech.

The 5K began. This time we ran south, toward Monmouth Beach and the base of the peninsula. Casey and Aaron were in full clown mode, hamming it up for the video crew. They did the airplane, swooping this way and that way with arms extended like wings. They ran backward, high-stepping and pumping their arms like parade marshals on heavy drugs. They did that giddy-up move where you imitate a rider on a horse by swiveling your hips to the side and shuffle-hopping forward with one arm holding invisible reins. They hadn't been able to do much training while we were on the road, so I knew that they looked forward to the moments when they could be a part of the 5k.

Feeling pressured by the camera's presence to show some spirit of my own, I joined in on this last antic—or at least tried to. The unaccustomed lateral scissoring of my legs provoked immediate dissent from my recently cramped hamstrings as well as from the tender tissue of my inner thighs, and I gave up the sad attempt at larking after a few seconds.

Lucy and Lily ran with us, Lucy completing her twenty-ninth 5K in as many days, while the three younger ones stayed behind to play on the beach. When we returned to the parking lot, Quinn stood there waiting with a high-five for every participant, insistent on not being left hanging by a single person. I felt glad for his sake that he had inherited his mother's sociability.

I had 9.78 miles left to run. A brief consultation with Brian, who had traded his Jeep for a pair of running shoes, resulted in a decision to cover the remaining distance with one long out-and-back. Once again, we began hoofing toward Sandy Hook.

Night fell. At our turnaround point, we had a clear view of the fireworks show on the East River. I stopped running and silently watched the pyrotechnics with my companions for a minute or two.

I wish I had experienced the wonder and national pride, but Angry Elf felt only disappointment. I had expected more: more immediacy, more spectacle, more crackle, and boom. It occurred to me that my underwhelmed reaction to the famous Macy's fireworks display was symbolic of how I felt at that moment about the whole campaign. Donations so far had fallen way short of expectations. I had serious doubts about whether the undertaking would serve as the springboard to future opportunities that I had assured Sunny it would. At times I felt as if I were sleepwalking through the adventure. Would I remember any of it afterward? Standing in the glow of the grand finale, I wondered just how much more I could take.

The next day would be Day 30—a day of symbolic limits for me. Thirty was my record for the most iron-distance triathlons completed in a single year. Thirty was also the record for the most iron-distance triathlons completed on consecutive days, set in 2013 by a handful of guys who stayed at a posh Italian resort and slept in the same comfortable beds every night. In Connecticut, I would confront these limits. With the way that things were going, I might also confront something more real: my personal breaking point. Then I would learn, for better or worse, what I had started this journey to learn: what, if anything, lay beyond it.

I turned around and grinded out the final 4.89 miles. As our little group approached BeachWalk one last time, I squinted into the darkness and spotted a cluster of people standing at the roadside. Drawing closer, I recognized my crew and family, including all five kids, who were awake and present to see me complete a triathlon for the first time since Day 6 in Nevada. I stooped down to kiss each child. I looked up to see the ground covered with chalk drawings.

"Did you guys draw me some pictures?" I asked as I looked carefully at each drawing.

"Sure did," Dolly said, "and our new friends helped us draw them."

I followed the direction of her jabbing finger and saw Rivers, who had been brought to tears by the sight of me swimming with one arm in Arizona, and who had since talked our mutual running shoe sponsor, Altra, into flying him east to support me for the remainder of the campaign. I gave him a combination handshake/hug, smearing sweat on his clean T-shirt.

Suddenly a passing car came within centimeters of grazing us. The resulting shot of adrenaline tore my attention away from my newest support and refocused it on my surroundings. I realized that our group was sandwiched between a low concrete wall and a busy roadway on a narrow shoulder.

"Let's get on the other side of this barricade," I announced.

My intention was to sidestep over it, but the wall was a little wider than I'd thought and my legs a little weaker, and I got stuck straddling it as though it were a hobbyhorse. Only by using my hands to lift my trailing leg and deliver it over the wall like a crane hoisting timber was I able to escape the embarrassing predicament.

I was well on my way toward becoming a man who was capable of swimming 2.4 miles, bicycling 112 miles, running 26.2 miles, *and nothing else.*

We filed into the hotel room, where I ate one of twenty-five cheeseburgers Kosta had brought from Barnacle Bill's and took an IV from Tina, the EMT. When the bag was empty, and the burgers were gone, our thoughts turned to Connecticut.

"Are you parked close by?" I asked Kosta.

⓭ ANGRY ELF

"I'm in the lot outside," he said. "Why?"
"Would you mind giving me a ride to the motorhome?"
"No problem. Where is it?"
"Right across the street."

INTO THE STORM

DAYS 10–16
KANSAS, OKLAHOMA, TEXAS, LOUISIANA, ARKANSAS, MISSOURI, ILLINOIS

I did not know that Kansas was in a different time zone than Colorado until I arrived in Wichita, after completing triathlon number nine, in Pueblo, just after midnight, on Day 10. So instead of starting my swim in the Northwest YMCA's twenty-five-yard indoor pool two hours late at eight o'clock, as I'd anticipated, I plunged in three hours late at nine. By ten forty-five, I was wearing my bike clothes and munching on a breakfast burrito outside the motorhome, eager to make up some time on the famously flat roads of Kansas. Alas, it was not to be.

"We need to get that blood test done today," Sunny called out from inside the RV.

Before the Fifty, David had made me promise to have a complete metabolic profile done on Day 10 (if I made it that far) as a precautionary measure.

"Yeah, no problem," I said. "But where?"

My hope and expectation were that finding a conveniently located facility and getting an immediate appointment would prove to be impossible and I would be free to get on with my day.

"There's a hospital right there," said Mike, a local guy who had come out to ride with me. He gestured toward a large building that was close to the YMCA.

"The CEO's a buddy of mine. I'll call him and see if he can get you in."

While Mike made the call, I did a quick interview with a local television station. The moment I finished, Sunny gave me the word.

"Let's go," she said. "They're expecting you."

IRON COWBOY

At the hospital, Sunny and I were ushered into an examination room, where I immediately fell asleep on the table with a needle in my arm. When the blood draw was complete, Sunny asked the doctor to call me as soon as the results came back.

"I'm afraid I can't actually release your husband *until* the results come back," he said as I snored on. "It shouldn't take more than an hour."

"Are you serious?" Sunny asked in disbelief. "He didn't come here in an ambulance; he came to get a simple blood test."

"I understand," the doctor said. "But if he left here and something happened that we might have picked up in his test results, the hospital could be held liable."

"Trust me," Sunny said, "James is NOT dropping dead in the next forty days, and if there is a hang-up with his body, I won't blame *you*."

I continued to sleep until the results arrived. Sunny then woke me up to hear the doctor's verdict.

"Well, you're severely dehydrated," he said. "Aside from that, all I can say is that you're the fittest person I've ever met."

I was now five hours behind schedule, and I knew nothing more about the state of my body than I had before the blood test.

The situation only got worse as I pedaled my bike through methane-scented prairie land to the west of Wichita. The strained quadriceps muscle that had forced me to walk the last part of the previous night's marathon gradually morphed into a sore spot in my left knee that would again force me to walk much of tonight's marathon also.

When it came time for the 5k, I was very pleased with how many people had shown up. Not only had they shown up, but some bringing gifts. One couple had seen Sunny post something about wanting healthy food, so they gifted us a fruit platter. It was devoured and appreciated. Another gift was an American Flag, given to me by a soldier who had carried that flag through Afghanistan. I definitely did not feel worthy of this gift and had trouble accepting it. He was genuine in his desire to give it to me, so I accepted it, and turned my head to avoid him seeing my emotion. This flag is displayed in my bedroom, as a reminder of all of the women and men serving this country, and the sacrifices they make so that my family sleeps safely at night.

Around midnight, the last few locals accompanying me in my slog around Sedgwick County Park went home. I still had more than three miles left to cover. Delirious with fatigue, I decided to take a nap before I attempted them. I crawled into

⑭ INTO THE STORM

the back of the van and asked Aaron (the only member of Team Iron Cowboy who hadn't already left for Oklahoma City) to wake me in one hour.

I walked the remaining distance alone, the desolation and darkness of suburban Wichita at three o'clock on a Tuesday morning mirroring my internal state. Just when I was feeling most sorry for myself, Sunny sent me a text message from the road, asking how I was doing. A childish impulse kept me from replying, wanting my wife to fear the worst, to suffer while I suffered.

When I finished, I climbed back inside the van and Aaron drove across the street to an open gas station, where we bought snacks and drinks and a bag of ice. Aaron sat next to me on the rear bumper while I ate and drank and iced my knee. There would be no shower for me that night, and the only sleep I got would happen during the two-and-a-half-hour drive to Oklahoma City.

"We're almost a whole day behind," I said. "I don't know how we can possibly catch back up."

"We'll see," Aaron said.

A surprisingly large crowd of nearly 200 Oklahomans, keyed up for the Iron Cowboy 5K, celebrated my limping arrival at Stars & Stripes Park after logging the first few miles of the day's marathon. I jostled my way through them like a sleepwalker; eyes fixed on a treatment table that had been set up outside the motor home.

"I hear you have a sore knee," said the table's owner, Rocky, a local massage therapist who'd come highly recommended. "Any other trouble spots?"

"My right shoulder," I said. "If you could focus on that and maybe tape it up, that would be great."

I laid facedown, and Rocky got to work while I dug into a plate of fruit and quinoa salad. It was a muggy evening, and before long I was marinating in my own sweat. Lucy and Lily came to the table and told me all about the trip they'd made to the National Cowboy & Western Heritage Museum while I was riding around Lake Overholser. Lucy showed off the cool sandals that she had bought.

"Can you ask Mom to come out here?" I asked her.

Lucy gave me a doubtful look, then shrugged and scrambled inside the motorhome. She was back within a minute. "She says she's not talking to you," she said matter of factly.

IRON COWBOY

I was expecting as much, because Sunny had been distant the last few days. My failure to respond to the increasingly concerned text messages she'd sent while I walked alone in Wichita didn't help.

After a while, Rocky asked me to turn over onto my back. When I did, I saw Sunny standing at the foot of the table, arms folded across her chest.

"Are you still mad at me?" I asked.

"Uh, yeah," she said.

"Because of last night?"

"Yes, and because you're nice to everyone except me!" she said. "You're nice to the crew, you are nice to the kids, you are nice to supporters in each state, but you are snippy with me and make me wonder why we even came if you don't really want me here."

Rocky seemed to be trying to make himself invisible.

"I'm sorry," I said. "I have been taking things out on you. Give me a hug. I promise I'll do better."

Sunny gave me a hug, but I could still feel how much I had upset her. She began to massage my feet with some Young Living Essential Oils, a ritual that I have always loved. I knew she loved me; I hope she knew how much I loved her. *I don't deserve this woman.*

As the unmerited pampering continued, I pulled out my phone and tried to catch up on the business side of things. With deep chagrin, I saw that Jordan still hadn't put a particular sponsor link on my website, despite the third reminder from me that morning.

You're nice to everyone except me.

Not this time. I sent Jordan a text message demanding the sponsor's contact information. He sent it immediately. Moments later, he sent me a photo of a television screen he was presumably watching somewhere nearby. It showed Game 6 of the NBA Finals. Golden State was leading Cleveland with 6:20 left in the third quarter. He knew I was a huge LeBron James fan.

"Glad you're getting to watch the game," I replied facetiously.

I then requested contact information for two other partners of the campaign who were angry with me for things Jordan wasn't getting done.

"Am I being relieved of my duties?" he asked.

"No," I wrote, "I'm just delegating them because you seem too busy to do them. I can't afford to get any more upset texts or emails from people saying you are not getting back to them. Clearly, your plate is full."

Rocky completed the treatment with a tape job on my shoulder that was so intricate and artistic I took a picture of it. Minutes after I resumed running in the sticky night, the intricate pink web became drenched in perspiration and fell off.

While Casey drove the RV south from Oklahoma City on Highway 35, Tropical Storm Bill was bearing down on Dallas, our next destination, from the southwest, kicking up wind gusts of sixty miles per hour and dumping as much as four inches of rain in some places. More than 250 flights had been canceled in Houston. The bike course that my Texas ambassador, Sean, had planned for me around White Rock Lake was now underwater.

By the time we arrived at the Life Time Fitness franchise, where Sean worked as a triathlon coach, he had decided to move the swim from the facility's outdoor pool to its indoor pool. When I had finished swimming, he'd decided to move both the bike ride and the run indoors as well. Just one look out the window left me powerless to argue against his judgment.

The wingmen hauled my CompuTrainer indoor cycling stand out of the van and set my bike up on it in a yoga studio on the second floor. I hopped aboard and started to pedal, observed by several local triathletes Sean coached as well as a few curious gym members who had no idea who the heck I was (beyond what they could glean from the Iron Cowboy posters that had been hastily hung on a wall behind me).

I noticed right away that the machine's calibration wasn't accurate. My power numbers were too low, relative to the amount of virtual distance I was covering. In other words, it was too easy. I made some adjustments, but they failed to correct the problem.

I stopped and explained the situation to Sean. "If I'm going to ride indoors, it has to be as close to riding outside as we can make it," I said. "What else do you have?"

Sean told me I was in luck—there was another CompuTrainer in the building. He fetched it and helped me set it up, and a quick test revealed that the numbers were right. All I had to do now was keep going for six and a half hours.

Three other stationary bikes were brought into the room and placed on either side of me for supporters to ride. A steady trickle of local athletes and gym members passed through the room to gape and gab. One of them was a friend of Sean's who had the same name but spelled it differently—Shawn—a once-and-future triathlete who was now more than sixty pounds over his previous racing weight.

"I see you've got a lot of wristbands," he said, gesturing toward the rainbow of rubber wristbands on my left arm.

"Souvenirs," I said. "People give them to me."

"We have one of our own," Shawn said. "We made it for our friend John. He died last year."

"If you give me one, I'll wear it," I said.

Shawn left and came back shortly with a wristband in royal blue. I read the inscription before pulling it over my hand: "SJW—Life and Determination—Racing for John Wadhams."

"What does 'SJW' stand for?" I asked.

"Speedy John Wadhams," he said, smiling.

"Tell me about him," I said.

In 2004, John was drinking and playing poker with some buddies when his host challenged the others to do a short triathlon the very next day. None of them were triathletes, or even in shape. All of them accepted the dare.

Early the next morning, John dragged himself out of bed and showed up at the race site, but his friends were nowhere to be found. John did the race anyway, finishing at the very back of the field, utterly miserable. He was hooked. Within a couple of years, John had transformed himself into a fit and experienced triathlete who dreamed of completing an Ironman.

In 2007 John registered for Ironman Florida. He was hit by a car while training on his bike and missed the race with a shoulder injury. Undaunted, John signed up for another Ironman but missed that one too, his shoulder still healing from surgery.

While preparing for his third attempt to reach an Ironman start line, John got engaged. His training took a backseat to the relationship, and the dream was postponed yet again.

In 2013, John attempted a comeback, but while competing in a short tune-up race in preparation for another crack at Ironman Florida, he started bleeding from a mole on his belly. A few days later, he was diagnosed with melanoma. John continued to strive toward his Ironman dream as cancer spread throughout his body. When brain tumors began to cause episodes of blindness during his long bike rides, he was forced to abandon his quest for the fourth time in as many tries.

Still, he did not give up. John signed up for the following year's Ironman in

🅮 INTO THE STORM

Arizona and trained as much as his illness allowed. At times he was so sick that he couldn't bike or run at all, only swim a little. Eventually, he couldn't even do that. On August 26, 2013, at age sixty, John passed away. Shawn and Sean were with John when their friend's Ironman dream was snuffed out for the last time.

"By the way," Shawn told me, "that's John's CompuTrainer you're using. He left it to the other Sean."

"No way!" I said.

"So thank you," Shawn said.

"For what?"

"For helping John do his Ironman after all."

As I continued to pedal away on Speedy John Wadhams' CompuTrainer, the trolls and haters on social media were busy denouncing my choice (which was hardly a choice) to ride indoors. They said I was breaking the rules, that today's triathlon didn't count, and that I had failed to do what I said I would do.

If these people only knew how badly they were missing the point.

As Tropical Storm Bill moved east, so did we. When we arrived in Shreveport at five o'clock in the morning on Day 12, it was raining sideways. By then, our Louisiana ambassador, Edward, had already called Casey to let him know I'd be swimming, cycling, and running indoors for the second day in a row. While we sat outside the Willis-Knighton Pierremont Health Center waiting for the pool to open at seven, Edward popped into the motor home, dripping wet. I was eating a bowl of Cheerios at the time.

"Cheerios?" he said. "Seriously? You're going to do a full Ironman on a bowl of cereal?"

"I eat all day," I said. "You'll see."

Halfway through my swim, I paused at the wall. A fit-looking woman with a Pepsodent smile bent over and extended a hand.

"Hi, I'm Sherri," she said with a southern accent.

I'd been expecting her. Sherri was a reporter for a local television station and a triathlete herself. While I finished the swim, Sherri watched the wingmen set up my CompuTrainer right there on the pool deck. Taking pity on us, she approached Casey and Aaron and proposed that I ride in her living room instead, mentioning that she had a pool for my kids to play in and a real-deal Cajun husband, Rufus, who would cook up a real-deal Cajun meal for everyone. We made arrangements to follow Sherri to her house.

A couple of hours later, I was riding in Sherri's living room, watching U.S. Open golf on her big-screen television while the wingmen finally snoozed on a sofa behind me. As promised, Rufus prepared a feast: boiled shrimp, red beans and rice, and other Louisiana culinary classics. Edward contributed spicy beef jerky and smoked chicken he'd picked up at Bergeron's Boudin and Cajun Meats.

I, however, couldn't eat any of it. Spicy food and James Lawrence don't mix. So instead I ate a huge plate of sliced apples, orange sections, and bananas; ham, cheese, and veggie sandwich; and four boiled potatoes with butter and salt that Sunny prepared for me in our hosts' kitchen. When I'd finished it all, I was still hungry.

"How about some Popeyes chicken?" Edward asked. "There's one right close. I'll get you the mild kind."

I nodded my approval. Thirty minutes later, Edward was back with three fried chicken legs and a surprise: fresh Bundt cakes in lemon, chocolate, and red velvet flavors. A taste-off was proposed and unanimously accepted. Then all eyes turned to me. "Count me in," I said.

I swallowed one big forkful of each, taken back by how delicious they all were. It was no contest; the lemon reigned supreme.

Sherri took journalistic advantage of my willing captivity, asking millions of questions and recording far more video than she could possibly use. I talked about the campaign's mission to fight childhood obesity, about the importance of healthy eating, and about the responsibility that parents have to set a good example for their children.

"Kids are going to eat what you put out for them," I said as I turned the cranks. "I don't know any eight-year-old who's going to grab the car keys and drive to the store and get a twenty-four-ounce Coke and a Ding Dong."

Sherri took a particular interest in the dietary aspect of my mission, filming Sunny as she prepared my boiled potatoes and the ZYTO team as they scanned the fingers of my right hand to determine my supplement regimen for the day. To my relief, Sherri did not film me eating fried chicken or Bundt cake.

More than once already in the campaign I had refused to let people film or photograph me eating. Hiding my consumption of junk food from the public for the sake of avoiding charges of hypocrisy seemed easier to me than explaining that I

⑭ INTO THE STORM

truly could not survive the Fifty without including some oh-so-delicious processed calorie bombs in my diet—but "don't try this at home." People were so gracious in bringing our family food. We definitely weren't going to turn our noses up because it wasn't good enough for us.

We transitioned from Sherri's house to a nearby Planet Fitness facility for the marathon. As soon as I got started on the treadmill, I discovered I was hungry again. We had passed a Smoothie King on the way over from Sherri's, and I asked Edward to fetch me a large strawberry Slim Blend.

It was nearly one in the morning when I stepped off the machine. I was hungry again. "Is there a Wendy's around here?" I asked Edward.

"Sure, what can I get you?"

"Chicken sandwich," I said.

"Grilled or fried?"

"Grilled," I said.

"French fries?" Edward asked.

"No French fries."

Ron drove two hours and thirty minutes from Springfield, Missouri, to Fayetteville, Arkansas, on Day 14 with the intent of participating in the Iron Cowboy 5K, and then going home. But when the 5K concluded, and everyone else went home, he took pity and decided to keep me company through the remainder of the marathon. Running alone with Ron through the dark was for me a bit like being locked in a bank vault overnight with a stranger who shared some common interests.

"Do you like to visit when you run?" he asked to break the ice.

"I like to talk a bit," I said, trying to offer just the right amount of encouragement.

Ron and I quickly found common ground on the subject of family. It turned out he had five children also, but his kids were a few years older than mine. I asked him for some tips on handling teenagers, and I tucked them away for future use.

Our course was a paved path that wound around Lake Fayetteville, each circuit covering a little more than five miles. The sun was up when we started, but had since gone down. As dusk gave way to dark, tiny glowing dots appeared all around us.

"What are those?" I asked.

175

IRON COWBOY

"Lightning bugs," Ron said. "You've never seen lightning bugs?"

"I thought I might be hallucinating," I said.

Ron had made a quick trip to a convenience store earlier to grab fruit and water to fuel the additional miles that he hadn't expected to run. After rejoining me, he offered to share, but I told him my support crew had me covered. When we finished the next loop, however, Jordan and Jessa were nowhere to be seen. Being the only members of the team who hadn't gone ahead to Missouri, they were on duty to support me while I finished the run. We set out on another lap, and I texted Jordan as I ran.

Me: "Where'd you go?"

Jordan: "Just up the street to grab something to go. You already back?"

Me: "Yeah, gone now."

We completed another lap. The van still wasn't there. We took off again, and at last, I broke down and ate some of Ron's food. I texted Jordan.

Me: "Where the freak are you?"

Jordan: "Pulling in."

Me: "Go to sleep and don't leave."

Sensing my anger, Ron left me alone for the next few miles. I tried to calm myself down by focusing on our surroundings. I only now realized that it was a quiet and lovely night. Moonlight danced on the water as a warm breeze caressed our skin. A mysterious upward drifting of the lightning bugs drew my eyes aloft. Now floating at the height of the trees that surrounded the lake, they looked almost like Christmas lights. Gazing higher still, I was awestruck by the vividness of the constellations.

For two weeks I had been living continuously in the imminent future—always trying to get the next thing done, to get today done and over. Now, suddenly and unexpectedly, I was fully present in the moment. Without premeditation, I stopped running, my eyes still glued to the heavens.

"Thank you for this moment," I said. "Thank you for this beautiful night—the lake, the stars, the lightning bugs. Thank you for my new friend, Ron. Thank you for the ability to run. Thank you for all the support I've received in every state I've visited. Thank you for my perfect wife, children and my team. Thank you for this journey, wherever it leads."

We started running again. Ron waited respectfully for a couple of minutes before he went back to "visiting" with me.

"Where do you hope it leads?" he asked.

⑭ INTO THE STORM

"Honestly, I just hope I can get an erection again when this is all over," I said. Ron laughed.

"Seriously," I said. "I worry about long-term damage—what I'm doing to my body. I'm starting to feel numb *down there* from all the time on my bike."

"But where do you *hope* it leads?" Ron insisted.

I thought for a moment.

"If people are still talking about the Fifty ten years from now, I'll consider it a success," I said.

When we got back to the parking lot for the last time, the van was finally there, dark and silent. The last several miles of the marathon had been rough, perhaps in part because of my earlier lack of fuel. I knocked on a window. Jordan slouched out and handed me a Styrofoam container with cold meat and potatoes inside. Seeing it, Ron wrinkled his nose.

"You know what's the best recovery food?" he said.

"What?" I asked.

"Blueberry pancakes."

"Really?"

"Trust me," Ron said. "Get your hands on some blueberry pancakes after one of these triathlons. You'll feel like Superman."

Twenty-four hours later I felt like Superman with a Kryptonite boulder on his back. I was sprawled across the backseat of my Missouri ambassador Ken's minivan, having just completed triathlon number fifteen. If ever I needed a miraculous regenerative food, it was now. Nothing, in particular, had gone wrong in St. Charles, I was just one day more tired, and one day closer to my breaking point. This trend could not continue indefinitely. I could not keep on tackling the same challenge with a weaker body.

Ken and his wife, Martie, chauffeured me to their home, located minutes away from the Katy Trail, where I'd run my marathon. Having seen the improbable quantities of food I had eaten throughout the day, Martie was quick to ask what I wanted to eat when we arrived.

"What are my options?" I asked.

"Anything," she said. "Eggs, steak, spaghetti, pancakes . . ."

"Pancakes!" I blurted. "Can I really have pancakes?"

"Sure, you can have whatever you like," Martie reiterated.

"How do you want them?" Ken asked. "Syrup? Strawberries? Chocolate chips? Blueberries?"

"Blueberries!" I said.

Martie and Ken chuckled at my childlike enthusiasm. What they didn't know was *why* I was so excited for blueberry pancakes, and I didn't bother to explain.

We entered the house through the garage. My hosts led me down a short hallway, through the kitchen, and into the master bedroom. Martie pointed to the bathroom and handed me a clean towel. By the time I'd finished drying myself off, I could smell the pancakes cooking.

I dressed in clean shorts and a T-shirt and sauntered into the kitchen. Martie sat me down at the breakfast bar and served me four fluffy hotcakes topped with a sweet blueberry compote. Before I stuck a fork in them, I asked Casey, who'd been napping at the house when I arrived, to take a photo for social media. It was meant for everyone's enjoyment, but there was one person, in particular, I wanted to see it.

After the meal, Martie showed me upstairs to a spare bedroom to catch a few winks before we left for Illinois.

"Sweet dreams," she said before switching off the light. "Let us know if you need anything."

Casey shook me awake seemingly moments later, whispering that it was time to go and that Sunny was ready to kill us. Right away I remembered the blueberry pancakes. Had they worked as Ron had promised they would? I took an inventory of my body. I felt exhausted, sore, and stiff, and the worsening blister in the nail bed of the second toe of my left foot was throbbing.

Oh well.

Wait, Sunny is going to kill us?

No one had notified her that we were sleeping at the house. She had woken up in a panic in the motorhome, wondering where we were and fearing the worst. I knew she would forgive us, even though we may not have deserved it.

When Casey and I blundered into the motorhome (which had remained parked at our staging area in downtown St. Charles while Casey and I slept in Ken and Mar-

⑭ INTO THE STORM

tie's home), we found Sunny awake. It was four in the morning.

"Quinn has a fever," she said.

"Bring him here," I said.

Sunny fetched our son from the back and laid him down next to me on the sofa bed. The last thing I could afford to do at this point in my quest was to get sick, and I knew the stress of the campaign had left me especially vulnerable to catching whatever might be going around. It was foolish of me to breathe my son's germy exhalations at such close quarters—but I didn't care.

It was Father's Day.

Casey started the engine and commenced the drive to Springfield, Illinois. When he roused me two hours later, the sun was up, and I noticed something I hadn't seen in the dark. Sunny and the kids had decorated, stringing up streamers and affixing butterfly-shaped sticky notes to the walls. When I peered closely at the notes, I saw that messages were written on them in the crabbed scrawl of young children. The nearest one read:

I ♥ your toenails.

I smiled. My toenails were looking rather hideous lately, one in particular. The kids delighted in their grossness, and I enjoyed their delight, little knowing that the grossest of those toenails would bring me to the brink of disaster the next day in Kentucky.

I roamed about the motor home, reading each butterfly message in turn. The next one read:

I ♥ your beard.

Like my mangled toenails, my mountain man beard was symbolic of the adventures we were experiencing as a family. Lucy loves the beard and hounds me whenever I trim or shave it. She sets deadlines and requires me not to touch my beard until I hit the promised deadline.

I ♥ when you laugh.

Lily, she is our laughing machine. I imagined Lucy and Lily laughing as she wrote this message. When the two of them get laughing, there is no turning back.

I ♥ when you play with us.

Dolly loves family time and is amused by the most simple activity. Little did she know, I love playing with her more than she loves playing with me.

I ♥ when you make breakfast for us.

Daisy. She is so efficient with her time and is up and ready every day without any incentive or encouragement from us. When breakfast is made, not only does her day shake out more efficiently, but she too loves spending time with the family, like enjoying meals together.

I ♥ that your farts smell.

Quinn, obviously. This little guy is incapable of saying anything that isn't funny. He has a great sense of humor, and spreads sunshine everywhere that he goes, just like his mom.

My family sprung another Father's Day surprise on me ten hours later, at the start of the marathon, when Lucy and Lily hopped on their bikes and vowed to do the full 26.2 miles. They made it until midnight and would have survived the last hour, I'm sure, but Sunny, having delayed the motor home's departure for Kentucky as long as she could, called them in.

I was not the only father on Team Iron Cowboy. Casey was also a father. He had left his wife, Ryanne, and three young kids back in Utah. The eldest, Spencer (five), had refused to speak to him since he left. Casey and Ryanne talked by phone every day, but some days the calls only made him miss them more. As Ryanne detailed her struggles, Casey was tortured with frustration at his inability to step in and be there for her, like he always is at home. He is a very engaged father, and he and Ryanne make a powerful team. Being apart makes teamwork very difficult. Our journey required a lot of work, but Casey managed to find small moments to play, to make it fun. This was much harder for Ryanne to do at home, and he felt guilty that he couldn't be there for her.

Things came to a head in their Father's Day call. Spencer still refused to come to the phone. Ryanne sounded more stressed out than ever. When they hung up, Casey broke down. Sunny was inside the motor home with him at the time.

"My family needs me," Casey told her.

Sunny knew exactly what Ryanne was going through on her own at home. She had ridden that same train, several times, through my other world records.

"Don't try to fix the situation," Sunny said to Casey. "You can't, and she doesn't want you to. Just listen, she just needs to be heard. She needs to know that you love her and that you are thinking of the family while you are away."

On its surface, the Fifty had only one goal. It was my duty to achieve that particular goal and everyone else's goal to support me in its pursuit. But the further we got in our journey, the more apparent it became that all of us needed to be there for each other. We needed to conquer every monster that came our way, together as friends.

⓮ INTO THE STORM

I AM THE IRON COWBOY

DAYS 30–32
CONNECTICUT, RHODE ISLAND, MASSACHUSETTS

I don't want to ride my bike anymore.
I don't want to ride my bike anymore.
I don't want to ride my bike anymore.

These words ran through my head in an endless loop as I pedaled along Beachside Avenue in Westport, Connecticut, a neighborhood of high fences, immaculate lawns, and pillared homes owned by the likes of Phil Donahue. The sulky refrain droned in rhythm to my churning feet, a mental counterpoint to my body's motions, but then, abruptly, the mantra mutated.

I won't ride my bike anymore.

I stopped pedaling and coasted to a stop at the edge of the road. My friend Chris, who had flown in from Utah to shadow me through Day 30, pulled over as well. Two local supporters, Jason and his wife, Linda, halted twenty yards ahead of us and looked back to see what was the matter.

I lay my bike down on a grass verge and stared at it like a frontiersman watching his horse die. Chris followed my gaze, nonplussed.

"What's going on?" he asked.

"I'm done riding," I muttered.

"You're what?" he asked.

"I don't want to ride my bike anymore," I said.

"Yeah, I get that," Chris said, looking around uneasily, as though for backup.

I coughed weakly and doubled over, bracing my elbows against my thighs and burying my face in my hands. A car passed, its driver perhaps thinking I had lost something tiny and precious on the ground.

With slow, deliberate movements, I dropped to my hands and knees, rested my butt on my heels, and lay my forehead on folded arms—a full-on prayer position. I wasn't praying, I was thinking about the forty miles of cycling left in front of me, and I was *rejecting* those forty miles, refusing them from the depths of my soul. Never before had I wanted so badly not to do something that I absolutely had to do.

An aching wave of hopelessness heaved inside my chest, and I began to shake. Snot leaked from my nose and blended with my tears as Chris loomed above me in silence; Jason and Linda made small talk at the edge of my hearing. Another motorist passed, this one slowing down to rubberneck.

None of these people existed to me. I was trapped inside my head with desolation as my only companion. I felt as if the very fabric of my mind were being torn in half by opposing forces—by the outright necessity of getting back on my bike on one side and my all-consuming desire to stay put on the other. Staying put was unthinkable, but continuing seemed impossible. What I *really* wanted was an escape from the whole situation: numbness, oblivion, anything but this purgatory of no good options.

Before the campaign, I had said in interviews that I wanted to find my breaking point and to see what I would do once I got there. Well, here I was. Now, what would I do?

Oddly, it wasn't any particular fiasco that had brought me to this point but more of the last straw. My day had started with an uneventful swim (aside from the usual shoulder pain) in a fancy indoor pool in Norwalk. Things soon went south on the bike. Pascale, my Connecticut ambassador, had planned out a four-loop course that toured the wealthy beach communities of Connecticut's Gold Coast along Route 1, explaining to me in her charming French accent that it afforded the only flat riding in the area. The problem, I soon discovered, was that stoplights dotted the road at quarter-mile intervals the whole way. Worse, it was Sunday, July 5, and the road was choked with Land Rovers packed with families who'd come out from their mini-castles to enjoy a day of sun and surf.

Our six-person peloton spent as much time stalled at intersections as it did moving. The others didn't seem to mind, but I felt a toxic case of road rage brewing. Approaching each intersection, I glared at the traffic light and willed it to turn green, or to stay green if it was already. More often than not, these telekinetic efforts seemed to have the opposite of the intended effect. I switched tactics and began to sprint toward stale green and yellow lights to beat the change to red, a maneuver that required a lot more energy on my bike than it does in a car.

Seeing how fast I was riding, my designated bike guide, Nat, who had been told I preferred to ride slowly, drew the wrong conclusion.

"I know why you're having such a good day," he said, smiling impishly as we stood at yet another red light. "It's because I'm the first Asian with whom you have ridden. I'm your Mr. Miyagi!"

I forced a laugh.

"I hate to burst your bubble," I said, "but you're not the first, and I'm not having a good day."

We completed one lap and started the second, and my mood continued to darken. I wanted to hurl rocks at the stupid stoplights and smash the windows of the stupid Land Rovers hogging the stupid road. I'd had enough.

"Get me out of here," I said to Nat. "Find me a place to ride where I don't have to stop every two minutes. *Please.*"

Nat's perennial smile flickered, as though I'd spat out the first bite of a special meal he'd cooked just for me.

"We can head inland," he said, "but it's a little hilly. Nothing too bad—just kind of rolling."

"I don't care," I said, "let's go."

Our group abandoned Route 1 in Westport and turned north on Highway 136. The hills came at us immediately. I would have described them not as rolling but rather as steep and decidedly more ascending than descending. I slowed to a crawl to keep my power output below the David-mandated 140 watts. Most of my companions rode ahead, while Nat stayed back with me.

"It'll flatten out when we turn onto Black Rock Turnpike," he said.

We turned onto Black Rock Turnpike. It did not flatten out.

"Huh. I don't remember it being quite this hilly," Nat said.

We passed through Redding and were approaching Bethel when I asked Nat to take me back to the coast. I had made a foolish mistake, allowing emotion to cloud my judgment. Was I choosing hills over stoplights? Had I lost my mind completely? My anger turned inward. I hated these leg-deadening hills, and my butt-killing bicycle seat, and the tropical heat of my forested surroundings, and the whole State of Connecticut, and everyone, directly and indirectly, responsible for my presence there—but I hated my reckless and self-spiting self even more.

As we came back toward the coast, the video crew picked the wrong moment to catch up to me in their rented SUV. Jacob, his face hidden behind a camera, shouted instructions out the window.

"Tell us where you are and how things are going!" he said.

"This is race number thirty," I said mechanically. "This is Connecticut."

I paused, distracted by a rash, self-spiting impulse to tear up the expected script and just vent.

"I'm pissed off today," I resumed. "Call me Angry Elf. Call me whatever you want. I want to quit!"

Saying this felt good, in a bad sort of way, kind of like scratching an itch until it bleeds.

"Everything hurts," I moped.

This was no exaggeration. On top of all my existing infirmities, I had a headache today. A headache!

"Nobody's donating," I grumbled.

There were other complaints that I wanted to add to this list, but a claw of raw emotion gripped my throat, and the only thing I could do was shake my head in an expression of all-encompassing disgust.

A few miles down the road, the SUV sidled up beside me again, and Jacob offered me a do-over, hoping my foul mood had passed and I would seize the chance to effectively tape over the image-destroying rant I'd delivered in the previous take. I showed him a middle finger instead. Jared, who was behind the wheel, knew me well enough to know I wasn't joking around and drove ahead. Moments later, I pulled off the road, dismounted, curled into a ball, and began sobbing quietly.

"Do you want to talk about it, James?"

It was Chris, still hovering above me. His gentle tone and earnest solicitude were irritants. I didn't want to be seen like this and said nothing.

"Do you need me to get Aaron and Casey here?" he asked.

I ever so slightly shook my head no. What could the wingmen do for me? What could anyone do? I was as isolated in my predicament as an astronaut left behind on Mars. *Something* had to happen next, but that something was a decision that was up to me. Whether I got up or stayed down would be determined entirely by what I was deciding to do.

A hand patted my back, more awkwardly than gently, like a toddler tousling a

⑮ I AM THE IRON COWBOY

puppy. If I were a dog, I would have bitten it.

My yearning for escape was so intense that I escaped in the only way I could—with my imagination. I pictured myself playing golf with my buddies back home in Utah. A couple of hours earlier, our cycling group had ridden past the Longshore Golf Course in Westport, and I'd ogled its lush grasses with a desperate longing, an almost irresistible yearning to pull up and play a leisurely eighteen holes. Within the past few days, my bike routes had taken me by an inordinate number of country clubs, each one pulling at me more forcefully than the last. Early in the campaign, seeing greens and fairways had been a comfort. Lately, however, these things had become a malicious taunt, a torment, and now here I was fantasy golfing in my head.

"Are you all right?" Chris asked.

My mind was a million miles away. I hadn't quit yet, but I was *imagining* quitting, what would it look and feel like to quit? It was vaguely soothing, like placing a hand on a wound. I took comfort in knowing my sponsors would be gracious if I packed it in, having expected all along that I would fail—though in all likelihood they would not remain my sponsors much longer. My followers, too, would be very supportive—and yet most would soon find other heroes to rally behind.

Before any of that happened, though, the first step would be to place a call to Casey and Aaron, who would pick me up in the Subaru, strap my bike on top, and ease me inside. They wouldn't say much, but their heartache and their undiminished love would be plainly written on their faces. When we returned to the parking lot back at the pool facility where the motor home awaited, I would slink through the door and break the news to my wife and children.

My family. My heart clenched as I pictured the faces of my five kids going slack in innocent bewilderment on hearing that daddy had abandoned his mission. I squeezed my already closed eyelids in a futile effort to obliterate the terrible image. Sunny, Lucy, Lily, Daisy, Dolly, and Quinn were the only people besides me who had been whole-heartedly convinced that I would succeed in my mission—partly because they did not appreciate its enormous difficulty as my doubters did, but mostly because I was their father. They had absolute faith in my ability to do anything I said I would do. After all, I had never given them any reason not to.

On the day before the campaign had started, Jacob had interviewed Lucy on camera, asking her if she thought I would succeed. "He can do it," she said, beaming. "I don't have any doubts. I think of all the crazy things my dad has done in his life, and I'm like, 'He can do it.'"

187

IRON COWBOY

This faith was sacred to me and was more precious to Lucy and her siblings than they could yet grasp. Their confidence in my invincibility gave them a sense of security and an attitude of hope and possibility that they naturally took for granted because it was all they'd known. I didn't want to see them lose that innocence. Perhaps it was inevitable that they would someday, but not now, not like this.

The hand that had previously patted my back now tried rubbing. It was all I could do not to slap it away.

The burning anger that had precipitated my meltdown slowly began to transform, the impotent rage of the bully's victim becoming the cool wrath of the relentless revenge seeker. The persecuted boy who's had enough, who's fed up and is not going to take it anymore was emerging.

No longer did I feel hurt and betrayed by the hills, the heat, my hemorrhoids, and all the other things that had gone wrong today and yesterday and the day before. I felt a new and icy resolve, a nothing-left-to-lose determination to defeat and defy the many causes of my suffering. No more hoping things would go my way. No more depending on factors beyond my control. I had a new attitude—or the beginnings of one—and the attitude was this: *Bring it on!*

"Do you just need a minute?" Chris asked.

I didn't hear him. His words were drowned out by an inner voice, a new and very different voice than the self-pitying drone that had forced me off my bike six minutes ago.

I am a robot. I feel no pain. I am a machine. I fear nothing. I am a beast. A monster. A superhero. I am the Iron Cowboy!

"Do you want to talk to your wife?"

Slowly, very slowly, I started to get up. Chris rushed to help, wrapping his arms around my chest from behind and lifting, but he was too weak and I too heavy. We nearly fell in a heap, and I had to do it myself.

Reversing my earlier slow-motion collapse, I got onto all fours, put one foot down, and then the other. I lifted one hand off the ground and braced it on a thigh, then the other, and then I was standing.

"What are you going to do?" Chris asked.

"I'll get back on," I said, scarcely audible even to myself.

"And then what?" he asked.

"I'll get back on," I repeated.

I wasn't going to make the mistake of thinking two steps ahead. There was no future beyond getting back on my bike.

"Are you sure?" Chris asked.

"Yeah," I said.

I got back on my bike. Having gotten back on, I decided to take one pedal stroke. Having made one pedal stroke, I decided to take another, and then another and another. In this manner, I finished the ride.

At the staging area, I sat down at a picnic table with my family and crew—including Brittany, who had just flown in—for a dinner of lasagna and salad.

I felt a shift in my identity, my consciousness seeming to crawl out of a mental bunker and stretch, catlike. Until now, the Iron Cowboy had been nothing more than a brand, a public persona. In the critical moments, before I got off the ground on Beachside Avenue, the Iron Cowboy seemed to have been born within me as an altered state, a version of me I could inhabit for survival when the chips were down. James Lawrence ate lasagna with the people he loved, and he broke down when his misery passed beyond a certain threshold, but the Iron Cowboy swam, biked, and ran, and he *would not be broken*—no matter what he went through.

I knocked out seven miles of the marathon before the Iron Cowboy 5K. I was just about to take off again from the staging area to attack the last sixteen miles with a few supporters when out of the corner of my right eye I caught a glimpse of Quinn, sitting alone and forlorn on the curb, sniveling. In his right hand, he held a small toy helicopter that appeared to be broken.

Instantly the Iron Cowboy became James Lawrence again. I went over and sat down next to my son.

"What's the matter, Little Man?" I said.

Quinn showed me the broken toy and continued to blubber.

I don't have many profound thoughts, but as I consoled Quinn, I had one. Until today, I had looked at my quest to discover my personal limit as a purely private endeavor, something that existed in a state of tension with my role as a father. When I actually met that limit on the side of Beachwood Avenue, when only the most powerful motivation I could find within myself would enable me to press on, it was my children who supplied it. In getting up off the ground *for them,* I had discovered that my personal limit was greatest, that I was my strongest and truest self, *in my role as a father.*

When Quinn was smiling again, I rose stiffly to resume running. Four hours later, Rivers and I toddled together, bare-chested and glistening, into the men's locker room at the swim facility to shower before rolling out for Rhode Island.

"That was a rough day," I confessed. "I really don't know how I'm going to do twenty more of these."

This was the truth. And yet, a part of me—an emerging part—*did* know.

I ran the last few miles of my next marathon, in Rhode Island, almost alone. Just one guy, Tom, a local triathlete, and coach, hung on with me till midnight. We circled an unlighted track at Narragansett High School using our cell phone screens as torches. There was little talk. But behind my outward silence, an inner monolog rattled along: *I am a robot. I feel no pain. I am a machine. I fear nothing. I am a beast. A monster. A superhero. I am the Iron Cowboy!*

The wingmen had noticed something new in me, I could tell. I was talking a little differently, in both substance and tone. *Don't worry; I've got this. Relax, I'm fine. Forget about it, I'm good.* I saw Casey and Aaron regarding me with reappraising eyes, like, *Who is this guy?*

Tom and I finished up with a lap and a half of filler around the motorhome, which we parked at a middle school. When he heard our voices, Rivers poked his head out the door. It was Casey's birthday, and all the adults were still awake, celebrating.

"Congratulations," Rivers said. "You just set a world record."

Kind of, in completing my thirty-first iron-distance triathlon in as many days, I had just surpassed the mark set by those guys at the Italian resort in 2013. It wasn't an official record, and although James Lawrence had once cared about this milestone, the Iron Cowboy did not. To him, thirty-one down meant nineteen to go.

"So where are you off to next?" Tom asked.

"Worcester, Massachusetts," I said.

"Wustah, eh?" Tom said, correcting my pronunciation. "It's hilly there. Good luck with that."

Worcester may be hilly, but the Nashua River Rail Trail in nearby Ayer is flat, and that's where I did all but the first twenty miles of my bike ride on Day 32. The smoothly paved trail tunneled between brilliantly green trees, crossing over the occasional covered bridge and passing a colonial-era stone church, serving up a delicious taste of the real New England.

Casey wasn't himself yesterday, and today explained why. He was sick, not just a common cold kind of sick, but sick and down kind of sick. He would spend the entire day sleeping in the motorhome. He and Aaron had compromised their immune systems by working their butts off for me, and only catching glimpses of sleep. Unfortunately, Casey drew the wrong straw and was paying the price and would spend his day wrapped in a blanket.

Three local stud athletes—Greg, Billy, and Simon—rode the full distance with me, having already swum with me at Indian Lake, which was so unexpectedly warm that I was forced to take off my wetsuit half a mile from shore, just about drowning in the process. As we approached each of the many street crossings that interrupted the eleven-mile strip of pavement we were cruising back and forth on, one of the guys would sprint ahead and check for traffic, then wave me through if it was clear, sparing me from having to stop unnecessarily. This bit of teamwork not only helped energize me, but also served as a bonding ritual for our group. I could tell it made the guys feel good to be doing something to lighten my load, and that made me happy that they felt useful.

With twenty miles left to ride, it began to rain, but the soaking only strengthened the atmosphere of camaraderie surrounding our little group, which now included Rivers. Somehow the two of us got to talking about music, and next thing I knew we were singing Garth Brooks songs—Rivers hitting all the right notes, me not so much. We belted out one tune after another, eventually landing on my all-time favorite, "Unanswered Prayers," country music's answer to "You can't always get what you want / But you will get what you need."

I couldn't help but reflect on Brooks' lyrics in the context of the campaign. So many things had gone wrong in the past thirty-two days; had they not, would I have achieved the goal of reaching my breaking point in Connecticut? Would I have found what I seemed to have found inside me at that crucial moment when I turned a breaking point into a possible turning point?

I was jolted out of my reverie by a sudden awareness that Rivers had stopped singing. I then realized that he'd only stopped singing because I had stopped. Tears were mixing with rainwater on my cheeks as the words soaked into my head and heart.

IRON COWBOY

We stayed on the Nashua River Rail Trail for the marathon. My Massachusetts ambassador, Monica, had set up a supply station at our staging area, consisting of a pop-up tent that shaded a folding table laden with food and drinks. At the end of each out-and-back lap, my companions (who still included the local studs) and I paused there to grab whatever we fancied. Around nine thirty, we finished our second-to-last lap and passed from darkness into the lantern-lit tent.

Monica leaped up from a camp chair to attend to our needs. My attention went straight to what appeared to be a piping-hot calzone sitting on a plate at the far edge of the table, away from the other refreshments. I made my way around the table as though in a trance and plopped myself down in the chair Monica had vacated. Her husband, Adam, was working away at a tray of chicken Parmesan at my elbow. I picked up the calzone, observed fuzzily that one or two bites had already been taken from it, and took a bite of my own.

Having taken care of the other runners, Monica turned back toward her seat with the intention of continuing her late supper. Our eyes met. Hers could not have registered more shock if she had turned around to find a grizzly bear stealing her meal.

Oops!

We headed out for the last lap. I don't know if it was the calzone, the energy I drew from Greg, Billy, and Simon, or the transformation that I had experienced when my body was peeled off of the grass beside Beachside Avenue, but I felt *terrific*. My body buzzed with pent-up energy, a cabin fever–like feeling that demanded kinetic release.

I picked up my pace a little. It felt good, but if a little was good, wouldn't more feel better? When we had covered half our remaining distance, we turned around and headed for the finish line, and I sped up some more. Greg, Billy, and Simon matched my acceleration without difficulty, but the others fell behind. I felt no guilt. My gut told me I needed this. For thirty-two days I had been swimming, cycling, and running in fear—fear of taking risks, of doing too much, of working too hard. I was sick and tired of holding back and I felt amazing as I ran full speed ahead.

I am the Iron Cowboy!

We covered the last two miles in less than seventeen minutes. My time for the full marathon was five hours and four minutes—equaling my best run time in the entire campaign (from Day 3). Moments after we finished, the local studs handed me a check for $1,600, having canvassed their athlete friends for donations. Things were finally looking up.

"I haven't felt that alive in thirty-two days," I told them. "My coach isn't going to be happy when he sees this heart rate data, and I might pay for it later, but right now—I don't care!"

One thing I had learned as an athlete was that sometimes what's bad for your body is good for your head—and the head's more important.

But I was right: I would pay for it later.

LIVIN' ON A PRAYER

DAYS 33–36
NEW HAMPSHIRE, MAINE, VERMONT, NEW YORK

In the nine minutes it took me to pedal my bike from Claremont Savings Bank Community Center to Claremont Cycle Depot, I was soaked to the bone under a dumping rain. On arriving at the bike shop, I paused my watch, something I did not normally bother doing when taking a short break from riding. This wouldn't have been worth mentioning if I'd remembered to restart the device when I resumed my ride with the handful of supporters that I'd just picked up—but I didn't.

I discovered my mistake some three miles down the road, and my stomach dropped. I was now faced with a choice between riding an extra three miles, so that my watch would show the full 112, or uploading incomplete data along with an explanation that my critics might choose to disbelieve. Then another idea came to me.

"You said you're riding the whole way with me, right?" I asked Jason, my New Hampshire ambassador.

Jason happened to be wearing the same make and model of watch that I use. What's more, he'd been with me all morning, swimming in the next lane over at the community center and guiding me from there to the Cycle Depot astride a sleek black Guru CR.901.

"That's the plan," he said.

"Well, now you *have to*," I said.

Minutes later, Jason's front wheel caught in the rail of a train track. His bike stopped moving, but his body kept going, launched clumsily through the air and landing inverted, then skidding a few feet on the slick pavement. I hit my brakes and rushed to him.

"Don't move!" I said.

Get up! I thought. *You're the only proof I have that I'm actually out here!*

"Are you okay?" I asked.

What if he wasn't okay? What if he'd fractured a collarbone and couldn't continue? I pictured myself slipping the watch off Jason's wrist and strapping it on my own, like a soldier rifling the pockets of an enemy corpse.

Bruised but unbroken, Jason eventually peeled himself off the road, leaving a fair amount of skin behind, and got back in the saddle. Almost immediately my concerns shifted from Jason's well-being and my precious data to the mountainous topography of Route 12A.

"These hills are killing me," I complained at the top of one grueling ascent.

Jason mumbled an apology, as though he'd put the hills there himself.

"Dude, seriously," I said after summiting another lung-busting climb. "I'm dying out here. Take me somewhere flatter."

"There is nowhere flatter!" Jason said. "Except . . ."

"Except what?"

"Well, there's a nice, flat ten-mile stretch right over the border in Vermont."

"Absolutely not," I said.

"I knew you'd say that," Jason sighed.

The next-best option, according to my ambassador, was a seven-mile stretch of road leading right up to the state line. We had just turned around to begin making our way there when Jason's wife, Audrey, came rumbling toward us in her pickup truck. She pulled into a small parking lot adjacent to a community baseball field, and Jason and I and the other riders with us followed. Audrey dropped the tailgate and laid out a spread of sandwich ingredients. Thankfully, the rain had stopped.

"What kind of sandwich would you like?" Audrey asked. "We've got ham, turkey, roast beef, cheddar, provolone, mustard, mayonnaise, lettuce, tomato, gluten-free bread, and regular bread."

She'd lost me at ham. Chronic sleep deprivation had rendered me incapable of making these kinds of decisions. When presented with more than one option for anything—meals, clothes, you name it—my brain froze. I stared at the sandwich ingredients for a long time, waiting for an answer to come to me. I tried closing my eyes for a couple of seconds to reboot, but when I opened them again, I saw the same unsolvable puzzle. Audrey's expression shifted from expectant, to anxious, to scared.

⑯ LIVIN' ON A PRAYER

Time continued to pass, almost audibly. *Tick, tick.* I felt intense pressure to speak, but the words wouldn't form. At last, after the longest thirty seconds in the history of the universe, I heard myself talking. "Um, all of it?"

It came out just like that—as a question. I sounded like a fifth-grader who hadn't done the homework, guessing wildly at the right answer to a question the teacher had asked him in front of the whole class, knowing it was wrong and already shrinking from the inevitable scolding. It was at this point that Jason stepped forward to rescue me, choosing items on my behalf.

We ran that day's marathon around an eight-lane track at Monadnock State Park. There is nothing in the world more mind-numbing than running long distances on a quarter-mile oval, but such venues do have the virtue of flatness, and my body—now paying dearly for my speedy marathon finish in Massachusetts—demanded flatness.

A spontaneous tailgate party broke out in the trackside parking lot as Jason and I and a few others went around and around like sufferers of some terrible obsessive-compulsive disorder. Lawn chairs and blankets were produced and put to use. Audrey dropped her tailgate once again, set out a tablecloth, and served up a home-cooked buffet of vegetable chowder, salad, and chicken enchiladas. (A special mild batch was put aside for me, the infamous spice wimp.) Entertainment, of a sort, was provided by Brian from ZYTO, who offered free nutrition scans, and by the owners of the Cycle Depot, who provided free tune-ups.

Somebody's smartphone was synced to a Bluetooth speaker. When I heard Meghan Trainor's "Dear Future Husband" blasting through it, I smiled knowing that my daughters, who are crazy for Meghan Trainor, must have been in charge of the music.

The sun went down, the moon came up, and the party continued. My surviving companions and I were completing what seemed like our one millionth lap when the playlist made a sudden change from Top 40 hits to something quite different yet equally familiar: a growling electric guitar riff backed by organ chords and a driving drumbeat—the intro to Bon Jovi's "Livin' on a Prayer."

I had no doubt whatsoever as to who was behind this one. Sunny calls it "our song"—an anthem for the no-safety-net, high-wire act, that has been our life together.

She said we've got to hold on to what we've got
It doesn't make a difference if we make it or not

197

IRON COWBOY

We've got each other, and that's a lot
For love, we'll give it a shot
Sunny, our children, the wingmen, and several others pressed themselves against the chain-link fence that separated the parking lot from the track, singing along. My group passed them just as the chorus hit—that soaring, infectious refrain that no human with a pulse can resist, regardless of how he or she may feel about 1980s hair bands.
Whoa, we're halfway there
Whoa-OH! Livin' on a prayer
Take my hand, and we'll make it, I swear
Whoa-OH! Livin' on a prayer
My serenaders smiled open-mouthed, and their eyes shone as they belted out these words. I felt the skin on the back of my neck go tingly. Our song had become *our* song: theme music for the motley pilgrim party that had assembled around my crazy dream, soundtrack to the beautiful, terrible journey that had united us and made us a thing apart from the rest of the world.

Team Iron Cowboy was indeed living on a prayer, pressing ever closer to our shared vision's improbable fulfillment, not by virtue of excellent planning, or superior organization, or logistical brilliance, but as the couple in the song, by the power of faith, love, and raw resilience.

Jason and I curved away from the others, and the playlist moved on. Just a few laps later, as my companions and I were cruising along the track's dark backstretch, there was a commotion on the grass infield just ahead of us, followed by an explosion of sound. The same group of giddy revelers as before leaped up from their hiding spot on the grass, Sunny cranking the volume on the wireless speaker, which she now held in her hands. The song again was—what else?—"Livin' on a Prayer" cued to the last chorus, where the band takes it up an octave. Our voices strained to match the highest notes, and yes, even I joined in the caterwauling. My heart ached with an all-encompassing gratitude, filled and bursting with the love and empathy expressed in this playful ambush. Never before had I felt such a sublime sense of group solidarity, of absolute oneness with a tribe, an extrafamilial "us." I caught Sunny's eye, and I knew she felt it too.

The moment passed. As the party wound down and my companions and I ran on in silence, I became reflective.

It doesn't make a difference if we make it or not.

🔟 LIVIN' ON A PRAYER

Before tonight, these words had never meant anything to me. *Does it make a difference?* Does it matter if we reach our goals or is it simply about the journey, regardless of the victory? I would not have started this journey had I not intended to finish; however, I choose both. I will conquer my goal, enjoy the journey along the way, with my greatest treasure, my family, by my side.

Everyone looked terrible the next morning. Brittany had the haggard appearance of being up most of the night. Casey and Aaron also looked more worn that usual. Casey and Brittany had taken care of Quinn, and his flu-related bowel crisis inside of the motorhome, in transit to Biddeford, Maine. There was a four o'clock a.m. emergency stop at a hotel, discarding my son's favorite pajamas in a ladies' room trash can. They had handled it all without ever waking Sunny or me, allowing us to continue sleeping without interruption.

Both Brittany and Rivers rode their bikes with me in a group led by my Maine ambassador, Jen. We churned out twenty-three-mile laps on smooth, quiet roads with views of a wind-tossed Atlantic Ocean. Jen had set up a SAG station at West Street Market, where her SUV sat stocked with food, drinks, and other supplies. We stopped there twice per lap (once in either direction) to refuel and use the bathroom. At one of these stops, Rivers sheepishly confessed that he needed a nap. He climbed into the back of Jen's truck, made his lanky body as compact as he could, and conked out. The rest of us rode off without him.

When Casey and Aaron discovered Rivers there some time later, they fell to the ground laughing. Then they took a photo and posted it on Facebook for others to laugh at and for Rivers to happen upon later.

I needed a nap too. The difference was that I couldn't have one. I warned my fellow cyclists that I was at risk of nodding off and asked them to keep talking to me. They obliged, but it didn't help. I felt sleep sucking me under with an irresistible gravity, a quicksand to consciousness.

I tried every little thing I could think of to stay awake: bugging my eyes out, squeezing the ends of my handlebar like stress balls. But nothing worked. Then, with no prior calculation, I blew air between my lips, making them flap and produce that nickering sound horses make. Instantly I felt the tiniest bump in alertness. So I did it again. Same thing. So I kept doing it.

Brittany was riding just ahead, creating a slipstream for me to cruise in. She heard the horsey sounds issuing from my lips and was first amused, then curious. "What the heck are you doing?" she called back.

"Keeping myself awake," I said.

"Is it working?" she asked.

"Oddly enough," I answered, "it is!"

This was not the first time that pushing myself to the brink of failure had forced me to become resourceful, to dream up an unlikely solution to a potentially show-stopping crisis. What I did not know, however, as I nickered along the Maine coast under hazy sunshine, was that it would happen yet again within twenty-four hours, and with more at stake.

Several members of the University of Vermont Women's Swimming and Diving team showed up at the parking lot outside the ECHO, Leahy Center for Lake Champlain in Burlington wearing bikinis and one-piece competition swimsuits. When I saw them, I quickly reversed the decision I'd made earlier (based on dipping my toes into the lake) to wear my full wetsuit and instead zipped myself into a sleeveless one.

Just before I waded in, I met Jim, an executive at Nathan Sports, my hydration gear sponsor, whose office was located a block away and who restored my sense of manhood somewhat by also donning a wetsuit.

"Your job is to keep me alive today," I told him, half joking.

Jim swam on my right flank and Hannah, the bikini-wearing president of the UVM Triathlon Club and my official Vermont ambassador, swam on my breathing side. Within 200 yards, the swim team had left us behind. The farther we got from shore, the colder I felt. A painful tingling sensation seeped slowly from my extremities toward the core of my body. My knees and ankles stiffened like rusty hinges. My arms became so numb that I lost proprioception and could no longer tell if they were moving correctly. It seemed as though I were swimming through a dense bed of chilled seaweed and soon my whole body would be entangled, helpless. With a flash of terror, I realized I was going to drown. I stopped swimming. So did my companions.

"I have to get to shore," I said. "I can't go any farther."

🔟 LIVIN' ON A PRAYER

"Are you serious?" Hannah asked.

"I'm freezing," I said. "I've got to get out of here."

"But we're almost halfway!" Hannah protested. "This is a point-to-point swim. Everyone is waiting for you at Leddy Park. If you turn around now, they won't know what happened to you."

Hannah was talking sense, but I wasn't making sense of it. All I cared about was getting out of the lake as quickly as possible, so without another word I started swimming back the way we'd come, forcing the others to do the same. I regained shore with what felt like the last dregs of strength left in my shoulders and sprawled faceup on the beach, slowly thawing out and coming down off my panic. Hannah approached and stood over me.

"What do you want to do?" she asked.

"Let's finish up in a pool," I said.

"That's not going to work. There are no vehicles here. It'll take forever to get you to a pool. Anyway, you've only got a thousand yards left."

Again, Hannah was right. If I transferred to a pool, I would fall so far behind schedule that we couldn't possibly get to Kingston, New York, in time to start the HITS Triathlon, the only official race I had chosen to include in the Fifty. I was terrified of getting back in the lake, certain that I would freeze solid and sink to the bottom if I did. I closed my eyes, tuned Hannah out, and racked my brain for a solution.

An image came to me, a sliver of memory from the very first Ironman that I ever did. It took place in a river that was so shallow that many participants—including me—stood up and walked portions of it. An epiphany struck me like a medicine ball to the chest. I leaped up and breathlessly explained to Hannah that official Ironman rules allow competitors to walk during the swim leg of a race if the water is shallow enough, and since I was creating my own courses...

"Whatever, dude," Hannah said in response to my rationalizing. "It's your show."

Good enough. I waded back into the lake until I was waist-deep and began to walk parallel to shore. My fear lifted, and the water no longer seemed so cold. I'd gone no more than ten or twelve yards when I spontaneously dived forward and began to swim. No big deal. I executed a few dozen strokes, stood, turned around, and swam back the other way. Half an hour later, my swim was complete.

The evening brought me back to the Burlington waterfront. Locals gathered and mingled with my family and crew at the parking lot of the ECHO center, where my day had started so rough and where the Iron Cowboy 5K would soon commence. I drank in the perfection of the setting, something I had failed to do in the morning. Sailboats bobbed drowsily on the lake's glassy surface, the gentle slopes of the Adirondack Mountains reposed greenly on the opposite shore, and I waited to receive a slowly sinking sun.

At seven o'clock I set out with a pack of thirty supporters. We ran north on a paved path toward North Beach Park, then turned around and retraced our steps. We were just over a mile from finishing when I saw a familiar figure shuffling toward us. He was a heavyset man of about my height with a mustache and a gap-toothed smile. I peeled away from the group, crossed over to the other side of the path, and gave him a double high-five.

"Way to go, Dave!" I said. "You've got this!"

Dave was the closest thing I had to a groupie. Vermont was the sixth state in which he had made an appearance. In the previous five, I'd learned his story in bits and pieces.

A Vermont native, Dave struggled with his weight throughout his childhood. Like any "fat kid" (his words), he paid steep social costs: always being picked last for playground sports teams, hearing snickers behind his back at church, staying home on prom night. As an adult, Dave continued to gain body fat and lose self-esteem. By the time he turned forty in 2010, he had weighed well over 300 pounds. He did not know his exact weight, however, because he stopped using scales after stepping on one and maxing it out—breaking it, in essence.

It was this humiliation that motivated Dave to commit and make some changes in his life. In 2012 he started riding a bike. Then he took up running. When an attractive woman who worked at the food co-op, where Dave shopped for the healthier foods he was now eating, challenged him to do a triathlon, he committed on the spot. He finished dead last, but he finished, and he felt good about himself in a way he never had before. So, he did another triathlon and another.

I first met Dave in Mobile, Alabama. He'd learned about me from *Back of Pack Endurance,* a podcast with a large following of people with stories similar to his own. During that day's 5K, the two of us recorded a short video on his phone to share with the *Back of Pack* community. No sooner had we finished than Dave fell behind and staggered to the line alone. Before he departed, he donated five dollars to the Jamie Oliver Food Foundation, despite recently losing his construction job and needing every nickel. I assumed I would not be seeing him again.

⓰ LIVIN' ON A PRAYER

But I did—the following morning, in fact, in Pensacola, Florida. Dave watched me swim in the bath-like Gulf of Mexico and then, while I pedaled back and forth along the strand, he climbed underneath our motorhome and put his technical skills to work, jury-rigging a temporary repair to the damage caused by our encounter with Bambi in Arizona. In the evening, he ran the 5K again and finished last again.

Ten days later, upon returning to the parking lot of Narragansett Pier Middle School, after logging the first few miles of my marathon, I spotted Dave in a huddle of Rhode Islanders waiting to join me for the Iron Cowboy 5K. As fate would have it, he'd recently gotten a call from a former boss who'd invited him to fly to Providence to interview for a new position. That interview took place on the very morning of my visit to the Ocean State. Dave tracked me down just in time to run his fourth 5K and finish last yet again. Then he canceled his flight home. He popped up again in Massachusetts the next afternoon and suffered through another Iron Cowboy 5K in New Hampshire on Day 33.

You might think that a person who always finishes last, yet who chooses to keep coming back to the start line, doesn't mind being slower than everyone else. That's not true. After Dave had fallen behind our group in Burlington, a familiar internal critic began to taunt him. *You're fat. You don't belong. Nothing has changed. Nothing will ever change.* But something *had* changed. Dave had gained enough self-belief through his efforts to give his life a new direction—and most recently through his six-stop ride on the Iron Cowboy Express—that he now had the strength to put a muzzle on that internal critic and tune his ear to a different voice.

Dave reminded himself that not so very long ago, he couldn't even run from his front door to his mailbox. Within the past few days, he had run eighteen miles and ridden a bike ten miles (with me, in New Hampshire). Having lost eighty pounds so far, he felt years younger than he had at his peak weight. Equally important, he *loved* running and cycling. Dave now shifted his attention outward and relished the beauty of his surroundings, the sinking sun spilling pink across the water, the dry air faintly perfumed by midsummer foliage and marine life.

Just then, Dave saw my group heading back his way. He saw my face light up with delight and recognition. In near disbelief, he watched as I broke away from the faster runners and came straight toward him to lift him up by word and gesture. The boyish, gap-toothed smile I got in return offered a clear window into how my new friend perceived the encounter. For once in his life, the captain of the team, the king of the playground, had picked *him* first.

IRON COWBOY

I said a final farewell to Dave outside the motor home a few hours later. Shortly before midnight, we rolled out for New York, Casey driving despite the fact that he would be racing the next morning and was still recovering from the same intestinal flu Quinn had picked up. An IV he'd taken earlier in the evening had restored him somewhat. Brittany had captured a photo of him making a funny face with the needle in his arm and posted it on social media.

It seemed like a good idea at the time.

I delivered my pre-5K speech on Day 36 in unusual circumstances, next to a Young Living–branded pop-up tent positioned right beside the HITS Triathlon run course. Participants working their way through the marathon passed in both directions as I addressed a gathering made up largely of men and women who had completed the sprint or half-iron-distance race earlier.

It had been another day of crisis and adaptation, beginning with a mad dash from the Subaru to the beach to avoid missing the official race start. I dived into Williams Lake a couple of minutes after the last competitor had left shore. Culminating in my decision to abandon the official racecourse after covering 31.6 miles and climbing 2,552 feet on my bike. I completed the balance of the ride on a relatively flat piece of road, guided by three local athletes who'd come out looking for me.

Midway through my speech, my audience burst into laughter, always a discomfiting event for a speaker when he hasn't made a joke. Following their eyes, I swiveled around and spied a pair of thickly bearded men approaching from the rear with the cadence of gunslingers. They wore speedos, running shoes, and tasseled leather chaps—and nothing else. Casey and Aaron had again raised the bar. I dropped my chin to my chest and shook my head in mock chagrin.

"Now that you've shown up in those things," I said after recovering my composure, "you're going to have to run in them."

A cheer from the crowd sealed their fate. The wingmen gamely ran (and danced and romped) their way through the 5K in their "assless chaps" (as they insisted on calling them, even though every cowboy knows that all chaps are assless). When they finished, their legs were chafed raw, just as I'd hoped.

Four hours later, I was lounging in the motorhome, feeling good about having survived another triathlon, when Sunny and Brittany burst in bearing a treat: sushi to go from dinner, that they'd enjoyed at a nearby restaurant while I finished the marathon. I grabbed a piece and popped it in my mouth, only to spit it back out.

"That's spicy!" I complained.

"No, it isn't," Sunny countered. "We specifically asked for not spicy."

She snatched a piece from the Styrofoam container and took a bite.

"Not spicy," she repeated.

"May I remind you that this is coming from a woman who carries a bottle of cayenne pepper in her purse?" I countered.

Brittany now seized a morsel between thumb and index finger and tossed it down the hatch.

"It's not spicy," she confirmed.

I opened my mouth to utter some withering rebuttal, but then remembered that Brittany, too, carried a bottle of cayenne pepper in her purse.

Disappointed, I ate an energy bar instead. Casey took the wheel of the RV, Brittany got down to the business of kneading the kinks out of my battered body, and I fell into a dreamless sleep, unaware that another Iron Cowboy scandal was brewing in cyberspace, the most determined effort yet to discredit my mission and destroy my reputation forever.

THE NEW NORMAL

DAYS 37–42
PENNSYLVANIA, OHIO, MICHIGAN, INDIANA, WISCONSIN, MINNESOTA

"Have you seen David's email?"

I had just finished an 112-mile bike ride on Route 209 in eastern Pennsylvania and returned to our staging area on the Delaware River to find my crew, family, and supporters rubbing elbows at the Shawnee Village Resort with a horde of cackling beer festival attendees. Sunny, though, seemed unusually sober.

"I haven't checked my email in two days," I told her.

"Better have a look," she said.

I pulled out my phone and scrolled through miles of unread messages until I found David's.

Sunny and James,

I regret that sometimes my communications bring crappy news. However, there is a serious issue to be addressed. The picture on Facebook of Casey giving himself an IV the night before a USA Triathlon–sanctioned event (HITS) is a big, big problem. This is a direct violation of anti-doping rules. Any use of an IV for recovery in or out of competition is doping . . .

It got worse when David reminded me that I had received numerous saline IVs over the course of the campaign and had participated in the same race, thereby violating the same rule. He urged me to release a public statement admitting that both Casey and I had unintentionally cheated. He also advised that we turn ourselves into the anti-doping authorities. What none of us yet knew was that some of my online haters had already reported Casey to the authorities and it was only a matter of time before they realized they could turn me in too.

"Does Casey know about this?" I asked, putting my phone away.

Sunny nodded yes, not saying a thing.

"What does he think?"

"He says he doesn't care."

This didn't surprise me. The problem was that Casey would say he didn't care even if he did; if he didn't care now, he would definitely care about it after the campaign ended, when he returned to chasing his own athletic goals.

I called David that night while running back and forth on a crushed gravel trail with a small group of supporters. The conversation did not go well.

"I'm not throwing Casey under the bus," I told him. "Go ahead with the self-reporting for both of us, but I'm not making any public statements."

"I don't think you're taking this seriously enough," David said.

"I don't have the energy to take it seriously!" I said. "I'm at my absolute limit out here!"

"I understand that," David said. "But you have to think long-term. What happens if you complete the Fifty and then get hit with a four-year suspension? It will discredit all you've achieved. You'll be just another doper. People will look at you the same way they look at Lance Armstrong."

"Let them!" I said. "I know who I am. I know what I'm doing and why I'm doing it. Nothing else matters."

I was looking forward to Ohio. My long-time friend Christian was the ambassador, and I knew that he would set up the perfect day for my crew and me. I had another friend living in Ohio, Grant. He and I became friends when I first moved to Utah. Tim had brought us together, and we had stayed friends ever since. I was anxious to see both of their familiar faces.

I had just started the second loop of my bike ride in Ohio's Cuyahoga Valley when a pair of cyclists passed our group heading in the opposite direction and abruptly U-turned. They'd been looking for us. I fell back to welcome the newcomers, one of whom—a little guy with freckled legs and a ginger-colored beard—I immediately recognized.

"I remember you," I said. "You swam with me in South Carolina."

His name was Christopher. He lived in Ohio but had been vacationing in North Carolina at the time of my South Atlantic swing. On the morning of Day 23, he'd woken up at four o'clock and driven fifty miles to Myrtle Beach to attempt his first 2.4-mile swim in the lane next to mine. Christopher had learned about me a year before and was inspired by my exploits to quit smoking, start working out, and overhaul his diet. When I met him, he was down fifty-one pounds and training for an Ironman. On returning to Ohio, Christopher continued to follow my journey, and he talked about me often at work—so often, in fact, that his colleagues teased him about his "man crush" and goaded him into undertaking a kind of dare when he saw me again on Day 38 in the Buckeye State.

It took Christopher several hours to muster the gumption to do what his co-workers had challenged him to do. Not until I was halfway through my marathon, and almost time for him to bail out to embark on the long drive home, that he cleared his throat and spoke up. "I have kind of a strange favor to ask," Christopher said as we ran together in a pack that also included a 6'8" Owen Wilson doppelganger.

"Lay it on me," I said.

"Can you sign and give me one of your speedos?"

Before I could even begin to formulate a response to this request, Christopher hurriedly explained its origin, suppressing the fact that the guys at work referred to my swimwear not as speedos but as "panties."

When we returned to our staging area at LifeCenter Plus, a fitness facility located in the small town of Hudson, north of Akron, I asked Christopher to wait outside the RV while I went in and searched for a spare pair of . . . whatever. I'd started the campaign with six Iron Cowboy speedos in two colors—magenta and kiwi—but at the moment I could find only one kiwi. If I gave those away, I'd be swimming in the buff. I went back outside.

"What happened to my other speedos?" I asked Sunny, who was manning the T-shirt table.

"I have no clue. They have disappeared into thin air," she said offhandedly.

Things were getting weird, and would only get weirder. Three days from now, in Indiana, I would run with a young man who, two days afterward, would have the Iron Cowboy logo tattooed on his back. In Minnesota, on Day 42, a pregnant woman would ask me to autograph her belly.

IRON COWBOY

I found Christopher and promised to send him a signed Iron Cowboy speedo as soon as I got back to Utah. I kept this vow and even sent him a congratulatory text after he completed his Ironman. Christopher replied with a photo of his right calf, on which the Iron Cowboy logo had been permanently inked.

I left Jean Klock Park in Benton Harbor with about twenty other cyclists and a double police escort—two beefy officers on motorcycles, lights flashing. We rode into a lush countryside carpeted in vibrant wildflowers bending in a stiff wind off of Lake Michigan. As a light rain began to fall, my supporters took turns asking me questions and sharing their stories.

"So how did you like *Minions?*" asked a potbellied man on an expensive time-trial bike when his turn came.

"The what?" I asked.

"*Minions.* The movie. I saw on Facebook that you took your kids to see it in Ohio yesterday."

I had *not* taken my children to see *Minions* in Ohio yesterday. Sunny had—and she'd slept through it. It had been an exasperating day for her. Sunny's entire morning had been eaten up by nuisances that included trying (unsuccessfully) to deposit the cash donations we'd been collecting into my bank account for later transfer to the Jamie Oliver Food Foundation and returning a shipment of Iron Cowboy T-shirts that had arrived in the wrong combination of colors and sizes.

All in all, Sunny's summer was not going the way it was supposed to have gone. I had promised her all play and no work, and she was getting the exact opposite. She hid her frustration from me as best she could, but sometimes it squeaked out. She had posted on my Facebook account mentioning her nap at the *Minions* movie as a bright spot. Sunny did not identify herself as the author of the post (no fewer than six members of our team had access to the account), but it should have been pretty obvious that it wasn't me. The man riding next to me here in Michigan didn't realize that it was not me that had made this post.

Realizing the mistake that he'd made, I burst out laughing. I pictured myself slouching in a cushy chair inside an air-conditioned theater, nibbling popcorn, and grinning at a silly cartoon, and I juxtaposed this image against the twenty-four-seven crisis that was the reality of my human-powered transcontinental barnstorming.

"Why are you laughing?" the man asked.

"I'm sorry," I said. "It's just that yesterday I started swimming at seven in the morning. I finished running at eleven o'clock at night. Then I stuffed myself in the back of a van to come here. It would have been nice to see that movie with my kids because I love Minions!"

Leaving Michigan, Team Iron Cowboy split into two parties that steered toward separate destinations. Jordan, Jessa, and I took the van to Muncie, Indiana, where I was to swim in Tuhey Pool, ride my bike south to Richmond and back, and then run around the campus of Ball State University. The ZYTO crew—Brian, Hannah, and Sariah—piloted the Subaru to the same place. Everyone else crammed inside the motorhome and cannonballed to Decatur, Indiana, home to the headquarters of Fleetwood RV.

Our flagship was in a sorry state. Apart from the front-end damage caused by the deer that Casey had hit in Arizona, the generator had been out for weeks, the pop-out side was inoperable, the extendable/retractable steps held together by a bungee cord, the fan belt shredded, and there were many other small issues. Casey and Aaron dropped off the crippled camper early in the morning on Day 40, backed the Mazda off the trailer, unhitched the trailer (at the request of Fleetwood's service manager), and barreled down to Muncie to support me. Sunny and the kids were dumped at a nearby motel with instructions to kill time until mid-afternoon when repairs to the motorhome were scheduled to be completed.

So far, so good. When she got to Fleetwood, Sunny found the motorhome right where the wingmen had left it. It hadn't even been touched, let alone fixed. At the service desk, they told her that they were too busy to get to it.

"Are you serious? We called you, and you said to drop it off!" Sunny said.

The receptionist shrugged her shoulders. She didn't care one bit.

Sunny's personality is such that she is always trying to help, and looks for opportunities to help. For this business to be so apathetic, when they knew what the circumstances were, was beyond what she could comprehend.

Sunny and Brytin, a Zyto employee, attempted several times to lift and pull the trailer through the gravel to reattach it to the motorhome. They asked standers-by and Fleetwood employees to assist them, and they outright told these girls "No." After ninety minutes, and frustrated beyond belief, Sunny finally shamed a Fleetwood service technician into lifting the trailer and reattaching it to the motorhome so that she could leave. It took him ten seconds; Sunny's irritation was through the roof as she climbed into the motorhome. The kicker was yet to come, because upon arriving at our staging area in Muncie, Sunny discovered that Tuhey Pool was the coolest, most kid-friendly water park the campaign had visited yet. There were waterslides, a snack bar, a two-story playground just outside of the waterpark and swarming with happily screaming youngsters. It was about to close for the day, and they had spent their day doing nothing, in an attempt to get the motorhome fixed- all for nothing.

"Mommy, why didn't we get to play here today?" Dolly asked.

Sunny turned away to hide her tears.

Around the time Sunny and the kids were burning time doing nothing, a terrible crash occurred within a group of supporters riding their bikes behind me through central Indiana. A local triathlete, Randy, lost control of his bike while descending a hill at high speed and flipped. He landed square on his helmet and came to rest face down with both arms trapped under his body. He remained conscious but had no feeling below the neck. Before an ambulance could get there, he began to struggle for breath. Knowing the risk they were taking, a couple of the supporters who had stopped to aid Randy turned him over to keep him from asphyxiating.

Randy was rushed to the nearest hospital and then transferred to a larger facility in Ft. Wayne. I was enjoying a mid-ride pit stop at the staging area when a few of the witnesses to the crash filtered in and shared the dreadful news. By then, Randy had regained movement on his right side but not the left. It was a greatly shrunken and much-subdued group that set out with me to get the rest of the ride finished.

Back at Tuhey Pool, word of Randy's misfortune was passed along in whispers to supporters arriving to run with me. As I stuffed my mutilated feet into my running shoes, I watched them deflate one by one, their expectant smiles and happy chatter giving way to grave expressions and silence. I stood and approached the waiting multitude. It struck me suddenly that many of them were unsure if the event would, or even should, continue. This took me by surprise; as heartsick as I felt, and as much as I wanted this ruined day to end, the idea of stopping had not entered my mind until now. Was it insensitive—or worse, monstrous—to keep going?

I pushed my way into the crowd, which enveloped me soundlessly, watching, waiting for a cue.

"Just keep moving forward," I said. "Let's go."

🔘 THE NEW NORMAL

I hadn't known I would say this until I did, but it felt right. Instinct told me that pressing forward would honor Randy and not disrespect him, and I wasn't alone. A palpable sense of shared purpose bound our group together as we loped around the Ball State campus. Many months later, when I reached out to check on Randy, who even then had only recently resumed running and still couldn't cycle or swim, I asked him if he thought I'd done the right thing.

"I've had some really hard days in my recovery," he told me. "I've lost hope sometimes, gotten depressed, but then I think of you. It's because you never quit that I won't either."

Approaching seven o'clock, we returned to Tuhey Pool once more for the 5K. I was grateful to have had my friend Joe with me. He had traveled from Utah to support me in Indiana, and this late in the campaign, the support almost moved me to tears. It was at the 5k start that I saw my wife and children for the first time all day.

"How did it go?" I asked Sunny, referring to her detour to Decatur.

"Fine," she said. "How was it here?"

"Oh, just fine," I said.

I could tell Sunny was withholding something and she knew that I was doing the same. The word "fine" had taken on new meanings for us over the past six weeks, becoming a kind of code or secret handshake. "Fine" meant: "*Not* fine, but I don't want to complain, and I *really* don't want to burden you with my complaining." It also meant: "We are in this together, working together, and our love brings us strength."

Around five o'clock in the morning on Day 41, approaching Madison, Wisconsin, something remarkable happened: I woke up on my own. Perhaps it was because the drive from Muncie was long (six and a half hours). Or maybe it was because the clock went back an hour when we hit the Wisconsin border. Whatever the reason, by the time Jordan slid open the van door in the parking lot of the Prairie Athletic Club, I was alert and even cheerful.

Waiting for me outside the van, huddled at a respectful distance, was a welcoming party of six Wisconsinites, mouths hanging open. Having expected me to blow into town with the pomp and swagger of a Rolling Stones tour, they could not hide their shock at seeing this disheveled drifter poke his head out from under a pile of musty blankets.

"Let's get started!" I said.

My Wisconsin ambassador, Annie, stepped forward and handed Jordan a binder with tabs labeled "Routes," "Maps," "Itinerary," "Madison," and "Contacts." She had put some time into this. Two local TV stations had sent camera crews to interview me, and a PA system had been set up on the pool deck. A local warbler sang the national anthem, at the conclusion of which I flopped into the water and swam to the beat of high-decibel club jams.

The music woke Casey and Aaron, who I had allowed to sleep in, partly as a gift to them and partly as a practical joke. I knew their first thought on finding the van empty would be that I had finally gone AWOL. They came running into the pool area in their speedos and, discovering me there, began to bump and grind like low-budget male strippers. Moments later, they climbed onto a six-foot balcony and executed synchronized cannonballs, competing for the biggest splash. Casey won.

A record 241 supporters ran the Iron Cowboy 5K with me that evening under a biblical downpour. (I know the exact number because Annie took a head count.) Standing out from the crowd was a petite fifteen-year-old named Ashley. When the 5K ended, and I set off to squish through the last several miles of the marathon, I was surprised to find her among the dozen or so runners who'd chosen to continue.

Ashley had started running in the sixth grade. Her parents, Mike and Jen, were not runners and had not influenced her choice of sport; she found it on her own. Very quickly, Ashley developed a passion for pushing her limits, racing as often and as far as her parents would allow. By the time she attended her first running camp in the summer before her freshman year of high school, she had run more than a dozen half marathons, and she pestered her parents constantly to let her run a full marathon. But the camp coaches counseled them to hold their daughter back, saying she was taking on too much too soon.

Mike and Jen were torn; on the one hand, they wanted Ashley to fulfill her dream of running a marathon, and the many half marathons she had completed hadn't seemed to do her any harm. On the other hand, the warnings of the experts made them hesitant.

Jen discovered me on Facebook around the time my tour kicked off. Seeing that I was scheduled to pass through Madison, an easy drive from where Ashley's family lived in Wausau, she made a decision. Ashley would run her first marathon with the Iron Cowboy. It was the perfect compromise, a real-deal 26.2-mile run, yet informal and noncompetitive. Mike could follow Ashley on a bike the whole way, supporting her, encouraging her, and, if necessary, rescuing her.

Before the 5K even started, Ashley had matched her longest run ever at thirteen-plus miles, and she was feeling it. When she stood up from the kneeling position she had assumed while I delivered my speech at Vilas Park in South Madison, her legs locked up. *I'm going to die,* she thought.

Seeing that Ashley was struggling, I slowed down to match her pace and silently willed her to keep fighting. With six miles to go, we paused at the staging area so I could duck inside the motorhome and put my children to bed. A minute later, Rivers barged in behind me.

"Ashley kept going," he said. "She said if she stopped she would quit."

We raced back outside and caught up to Ashley as quickly as possible. Her formerly graceful stride had degenerated into the wounded reeling of a buckshot turkey. She was fighting back the tears.

How young is too young to run a marathon? To how much suffering should a young athlete be allowed to be subjected? These are important questions, but not questions I spend a lot of time thinking about because I've seen more lives soured by risking too little than by risking too much. Achieving success of any kind in life demands resilience. Like physical fitness, this kind of mental fitness cannot be purchased into a bottle but must be developed through consistent effort over an extended period of time. I began to cultivate my mental fitness at age eleven when I took up wrestling, and I've never regretted it. Another person in my place might have urged caution on Ashley, offered her a way out. I did not.

"Keep pushing," I told her as we entered the last mile. "There's a better you on the other side of that finish line, I promise."

As we approached the finish line, the other runners backed off, allowing Ashley to fulfill her dream alone with me. We held clasped hands aloft as we took the final stride and then embraced while our companions cheered. The tears she'd been holding back burst forth, but she was smiling now, no longer grimacing.

After the usual business of hugs, photographs, and farewells, Annie's friend Nettie led me to a pop-up tent where I grabbed a quick meal of quinoa salad, scalloped potatoes, and turkey wraps. I then slipped into the front passenger seat of her crossover SUV, and she drove me a couple of miles to an Anytime Fitness center in downtown Madison, where she had arranged for me to take a shower. We parked in a deserted underground garage and rode an elevator to the third floor.

"So what's your story, Nettie?" I asked, partly because I was curious but mostly because riding in an elevator in silence with someone you've just met is awkward.

"The elevator version?" she laughed. "I've lost 106 pounds in the past two years."

The full story was this: Nettie just woke up one morning and decided she was sick and tired of having a body that didn't match her "adventurous, sporty, fun, and sassy" personality. She cleaned up her diet and took up swimming and running, and the pounds came flying off. By the time I met her, she had run three marathons and opened up her personal training and nutrition coaching business.

But the biggest change Nettie had experienced wasn't physical. "Before I took control of my life, I had small dreams and big limitations," she told me. "Now I have big dreams and no limitations."

Twenty minutes later, Nettie and I got back in the car and crept up to the gate. She put her ticket into the machine, and the gate lifted, as did a sliding metal door that stood well behind the gate at the top of a steep ramp.

"Oh, crap!" I said. "I left my phone in the bathroom!"

"No problem," Nettie said.

She reversed, swung the car around, and pulled into the same parking spot that we'd just left. I took a second elevator ride and found my phone where I had left it on the bathroom sink. When we returned to the gate, Nettie realized she no longer had an exit ticket.

There was a "Help" button on the machine. She pressed it. No answer.

"I'll just get a new ticket," Nettie said. "Wait here."

She turned off the car and climbed out, hiked to the top of the ramp, and exited the garage through a pedestrian door next to the sliding metal door. It was eleven thirty. I thought, *Well, this kind of sucks.*

Hungry again, I checked the backseat and discovered a large carton of fresh cherries. As I worked my way through them, I pulled out my phone and checked my email. I skipped the business-related ones, which Sunny would handle, and opened one from my Aunt Janice.

James;

Many days have passed, & I have written this e-mail over & over in my mind. Words r not able to express what I feel inside . . . for example, whenever I am talking to some1 about what/why u r doing what u r doing, I get sooo excited! Just be4 u embarked on this amazing adventure, I finally got the 'click,' &

understood.

However, as I've followed your journey (spend hrs/day), I've gained a new understanding + respect.

Anyway, I just wanted u to know, u r special!

WOOT WOOT . . . go get 'em cowboy!

Hugs J

My mother's half-sister Janice was only twenty-four years old in 1990 when she suffered a major stroke. It left her completely paralyzed, unable to walk, talk, eat, or bathe herself, but her intellectual faculties were unaffected. She composed emails with the aid of special glasses that used a laser to link her eye movements to a virtual keyboard on a computer screen. I knew how slow and tedious this process was for Aunt Janice, and most of the messages I got from her were just a few words in length. Writing this one must have been as exhausting for her as completing my forty-first triathlon in forty-one days was for me.

Suddenly, it no longer bothered me that I was trapped inside a parking garage at almost midnight, facing a five-hour drive to Waconia, Minnesota, and another triathlon the next day.

I looked up from my phone and saw Nettie's face through a glass panel in the door she'd exited, mouthing my name soundlessly. The door itself shivered in recoil to the pounding of her fists. I got out of the car, walked up the ramp, and opened the door.

"Don't let it close behind you!" she said. "It's locked."

"Did you get another ticket?"

"The machine wouldn't give me one. It knows I'm not a car."

I gestured for Nettie to take hold of the door and went over to the ticket machine to try it out for myself. She was right.

"I'll flag someone down," I said.

I stepped out onto University Avenue and waved my arms overhead at the next approaching car, which kept going.

"It's not going to work," Nettie said. "They'll think you're a crazy homeless person."

I looked at myself. I was wearing lime green shorts and running shoes, no shirt. I had a grizzled beard, prison-yard muscles, and tattoos everywhere. She was right.

"I'll just have to call Annie," Nettie sighed.

She called Annie and told her she was trapped inside a parking garage with the Iron Cowboy.

"How is that even possible?" Annie asked.

Minutes later, Annie arrived in her car and got a new ticket at the entrance. Then came the hard part; we had to get both cars through the exit gate and the sliding door in one go. Nettie pulled right up to Annie's rear bumper.

"You'd better switch to Annie's car," Nettie said, "in case I don't make it."

Both cars made it through, barely. Annie drove me back to the staging area to reunite with my family and crew while Nettie drove home. On the way, Nettie reached into the backseat for the carton of fresh cherries she had bought for herself in the morning. She found the cartoon but no cherries. Only the pits remained.

At two o'clock in the afternoon on Day 42, my Minnesota ambassador, Christina, received a phone call from Casey, who requested that she arrange to move the swim she had planned for me in Lake Waconia to a pool, explaining that my shoulder injury made open-water swimming inadvisable. Christina had sixteen hours to find a new venue and share the revised plan with the kayakers and other volunteers she'd recruited to help out, as well as with the press and the local endurance community.

When I stepped out of the RV and onto the parking lot at Life Time Fitness in Chanhassen, Christina immediately introduced me to a pair of physical therapists from TRIA Orthopaedic Center, who offered to massage my shoulder, tape it up—whatever I needed—but I declined. By this point in the campaign, I had come to accept that nothing helped and the problem just wasn't going to get any better. Focusing on what I could control, I had evolved an asymmetrical swim style that combined full strokes with my left arm and half strokes with the other, an inelegant but workable compromise between the competing objectives of pain management and efficiency.

I completed the swim in one hour, twenty minutes, and forty-seven seconds, a pleasant surprise, as my recent swims had been running closer to ninety minutes. Only after I had climbed out of the water and toweled off did I realize that, as in Washington, my watch had been on the wrong setting and I'd inadvertently swum 4,224 yards instead of 4,224 meters. So I got back in the pool for another thirteen minutes of abuse. I then moved to the hot tub to warm up. Rivers soaked with me.

"I can't even describe how excruciating this is," I said to him. "The swim is still the hardest part of the entire day, every day."

To underscore the point, I winged my right arm out to the side, elbow bent. When it reached an angle of seventy degrees, I felt a sharp jolt of pain, winced, and let the arm drop.

"I can't even lift a fork to my mouth," I added, with a hint of pride.

"When I saw you in Flagstaff you were swimming with one arm," Rivers said. "It must be a *little* better."

"Nothing has changed," I insisted. "The only difference is that I just stopped complaining about it."

In fact, I'd also stopped *thinking* about it. Weeks before, the pain I endured each morning in the water had dominated my consciousness from the first stroke to the last. Now it was background noise. After forty-one days, my mind seemed to have adapted to the new "normal" of exercising fourteen hours out of every twenty-four and sleeping on the floor of a van. I had found a kind of equilibrium in the Fifty lifestyle, not by overcoming weariness and discomfort, which were as constant and severe as ever, but by developing the capacity to ignore these things, to direct my attention elsewhere.

I am a robot. I am a machine.

More than one hundred Minnesotans rode their bikes with me through the blazing heat on the Dakota Regional Trail on the north side of Lake Waconia. Four hours in, Rivers called out to me from a few bike lengths behind.

"So what do you want to do tomorrow?" he asked, louder than necessary.

"Oh, I don't know," I shouted back. "I was thinking maybe . . . another Ironman?"

Our companions laughed, unaware that Rivers and I trotted out this routine almost daily. It was our way of having fun with the idea that swimming, cycling, and running 140.6 miles every day had indeed become normal. There was more than a trace of cockiness in the gag. With eight and a half days left to go, I felt nothing short of an act of God, a lightning strike or a twister, could stop me from reaching the ultimate finish line in Utah.

I completed the marathon around eleven. Sunny's cousin, Mike, had come from Utah, and had run the entire marathon with me. He had never run that far, and was only trained with basic run fitness. It nearly killed him, but he continued to fight and finish that whole marathon with me. He checked back with me later that night to let me know that he was back at his hotel, and that he was feeling much better than when he had finished. I was impressed, no doubt about it!

I crept inside the motorhome, where I found my five children lined up like matchsticks on the master bed, their cherubic faces slack with sleep, and my love became a physical thing, an almost painful swelling in the chest. Moments later, a thunderstorm hit. Minutes after we rolled out for Iowa, a tornado ripped through Minnesota.

The irony was not lost on me.

⑰ THE NEW NORMAL

CARNIVAL OF SWEAT

DAYS 43–47
IOWA, NEBRASKA, SOUTH DAKOTA, NORTH DAKOTA, MONTANA

A faint chill rose off the water rippling at my feet. Head bowed, I contemplated the pale blue fluid in the way a six-year-old might regard a lump of steamed spinach on his dinner plate. Hazy morning sunshine warmed my back pleasantly, heightening the contrast between my present comfort and looming discomfort, feeding my reluctance to take the plunge.

Splashing sounds drew my attention toward the opposite side of the pool, where the only other swimmers present—three or four teenage girls—were crowded together for some unknown reason.

Okay, jump! I did not jump. *One, two, three, go!* Again I disobeyed my mental command. It was the same every morning. This ritual hesitation had become the symbolic low point of a day in the life of the Iron Cowboy—not the struggle itself but the dread of it.

The end was always the same too. My mind went blank. I felt my lungs fill with air. I fell in.

Two hours later, now dressed in my cycling kit, I returned to the deck of the Mason City Aquatic Center's outdoor pool from the motorhome to fill up on a hot breakfast that Cathy, my Iowa ambassador, had prepared. As I made my way toward the steaming spread, I was approached by a nervous-looking girl of fifteen or sixteen who wore a blindingly bright, multicolored swimsuit. In her right hand was a single piece of paper currency, which she held out toward me as one might offer a hunk of meat to a wild predator.

"Excuse me, Mr. Cowboy," she said, blushing. "I found this on the bottom of the pool when I was swimming. I want to donate it to your charity."

"Wait, did you come here for me?" I asked surprised.

"Yes, my friends and I," she said.

"Then why did you swim at the other end of the pool?"

"We didn't want to bother you."

"Bother me?" I said. "Nonsense!"

I handed my phone to Casey, and he snapped a photo of me with one hand on my shy young supporter's shoulder and the other showing off her donation. All I needed now was for 94,000 other generous supporters to discover a ten-dollar bill on the bottom of a pool and I would achieve my fund-raising goal.

I filled a paper plate with scrambled eggs, country potatoes, bacon, and watermelon chunks and sat down at a shaded metal table with Sunny, the wingmen, and Dallas, who had rejoined the campaign in Minnesota. The rest of our family, the crew, and the few people who had shown up to ride with me, occupied surrounding tables. We dug in with gusto, but after a minute or two my tablemates fell silent, and their chewing slowed.

"This bacon taste like soap," Casey said with a crooked smile.

"They do!" Aaron said laughing. "Dish soap!"

They kept eating them, snickering with each crunch. The bacon did taste like soap. I too kept eating.

The classic postcard image of Iowa depicts a straight, flat country road bordered by windswept fields of man-high corn. That's where I rode my bike on Day 43. I knew as soon as I set out with six supporters that my two-wheeled journey through Northern Iowa would be one of those long stare-downs between sleepiness and willpower. The last time I had felt like I was losing the battle of staying awake (and upright) on my bike was in Maine. I asked my companions to keep me alert by engaging me in conversation. The only problem with this idea was that I didn't actually feel like talking.

"So what do you eat?" asked Joe, a firefighter from Waterloo.

"Food," I answered. (Boy, was I tired of that question.)

"What kind of food?" Joe asked, unfazed by my surliness.

"Whatever they put in front of me," I said.

Joe took his cue and fell silent. I felt guilty.

"Do you have a family?" I asked.

"I do," Joe said, reanimated. "I have a wife and three children, two girls and a boy. The youngest was born six weeks ago."

Forty miles down the road, I was still wrestling against slumber and still seeking aid in that struggle from those around me, who took turns enduring stilted, one-sided conversations with the supposed star of the show. When Joe's turn came back around, I made an effort to be nicer.

"Do you have a family?" I asked.

Joe turned his head and studied me, trying to determine if I was pulling his leg. I was not. I had no memory of asking him the same question previously. Six weeks of sleep deprivation had turned my brain to mush.

"I do," Joe said patiently. "I have a wife and three children, two girls and a boy. The youngest was born six weeks ago."

At the next refueling stop, I pulled Rivers aside. "I'm really struggling today," I told him. "I need some help."

"Just eat some food and keep riding," he said.

Just the help that I needed—a blunt reminder that nobody *could* do anything for me. My supporters were already doing everything in their power to lighten my load: riding their bikes in front of me to break the wind and keeping me well supplied with food and drink, but staying awake was a job I had to do for myself. I knew my nemesis would blink eventually; it always did. I just had to outlast it.

We got back on our bikes. Approaching one hundred miles, I found Joe once again on my left shoulder.

"Do you have a family?" I asked him.

This time he laughed. "I do," he said. "I have a wife and three children, two girls and a boy. The youngest was born six weeks ago."

"I think I asked you that before," I said.

"Three times!" Joe said, laughing again.

Despite my embarrassment, I took it as a good sign that at least I now remembered having asked the same question before, whereas earlier I had not. Sleep had lost the day's game of chicken. I would survive to face it again the next day.

With a few laps left in my Day 44 swim at the Cooper YMCA in Lincoln, Nebraska, my lone companion hoisted himself out of the pool, dashed across the deck through a light rain, and vomited noisily into a garbage can. I took perverse satisfaction in the spectacle, judging that no one could better appreciate what I was achieving than a person who tried to complete a single leg, just one, of my triathlons and failed.

Fifteen supporters started the bike ride with me—more than I had expected in Nebraska, but not all of them were Nebraskans. The longer the campaign wore on, the further people traveled to support me. A guy named Brian, from Ohio, had joined up with us in Indiana and stayed on through yesterday's triathlon in Iowa. Today's group included a woman from Kansas City, Kim, who had made the long drive to Lincoln to draw inspiration for her battle with breast cancer.

About thirty miles in, we were joined by four more cyclists. Among them was an Iowan named Therese, whose voice shook with emotion when I welcomed her. "I can't believe it!" she said. "I'm riding with the Iron Cowboy!"

This was happening more and more as we pressed westward—people reacting to meeting me the way I might react to meeting LeBron James. Smiling from ear to ear, Therese accelerated hard to position herself in front of me and provide a helpful pull, but then she forgot to slow down. My power output leaped by twenty watts in the effort to latch on to her back wheel.

"So, what do you eat, anyway?" Therese called back, swiveling her head around dangerously as she spoke.

"Eyes on the road, please," I said.

Near the end of the ride, I heard a hubbub behind me—first laughter, then the sound of men imitating women's voices, rather badly, as in a *Monty Python* skit. Moments later, Casey pulled up alongside me on his bike, wearing a turquoise party dress and a long, blond wig under his helmet. Right behind him came Aaron, clad in a satin number with a floral pattern and the twin to Casey's headpiece.

"Riding a bike 112 miles?" Casey scowled, using Jimmy Fallon impersonation of a teenage girl. "Ew!"

"I just *love* the Iron Cowboy!" Aaron followed in a crackling falsetto. "I'm gonna marry him!"

In recent days, the campaign had taken on a carnivalesque atmosphere. Superfan freakouts, multi-state supporters, swelling 5K turnouts, increasing media interest, and an exploding social media following (people were starting to see that I might actually pull this thing off) were all the significant contributors to this traveling circus vibe. Wingman hijinks—now a daily occurrence—was another. Silly and playful in a spontaneous way from the beginning, Casey and Aaron had since matured (if that's the word) into quasi-professional jokers, devoting more energy than seemed sane to planning stunts intended to surprise and amuse me.

In Madison, they had crashed my 5K speech wearing body paint and little else. In Minnesota, they rolled past me on a borrowed tandem bike attired in Iron Cowboy racing uniforms complete with aerodynamic helmets. (It was the juxtaposition of these space-age brain buckets and the wingmen's survivalist beards that elevated the image from merely amusing hilariousness.) Now here they were rocking thrift store shifts and wigs my daughters had bought at the dollar store.

I couldn't help but wonder what these guys had lined up for me tomorrow. I actually found myself looking forward to the next day's triathlon just a bit more than I would have done otherwise.

I didn't have to wait long to learn what Casey and Aaron's next trick would be. A few minutes into my indoor pool swim at Sanford Wellness Center in Sioux Falls, South Dakota, a pair of six-foot sharks began to circle me. The wingmen had improvised dorsal fins using cardboard, silver spray paint, and bungee cords. It took all of thirty seconds for the cardboard to soak through and turn limp.

Not every trick can be the best trick.

My South Dakota ambassador, Brian, had planned a bike ride for me that would take place entirely on the Big Sioux River Recreation Trail and Greenway, which was accessible, right outside the Sanford Wellness Center. Flat, smooth, and free of stops, it was perfectly suited to the low-energy kind of riding I liked, unless it was windy, and it's always windy in South Dakota.

My four companions and I rolled out of the parking lot together, made a right turn onto the trail, and ran smack into sustained winds of twenty-five to thirty miles per hour. A high school kid on a mountain bike packed it in after ten miles. I didn't have that option. The best I could do was tuck in behind my friend Shad, fresh in from Utah, or another cyclist. Even with the help, I felt as though I were riding on two flat tires, getting nothing for my effort.

Fortunately, I had something to take my mind off the wind. Unfortunately, that something was extreme discomfort in and around my rear end. The situation in these sensitive parts of my body had not improved since initially reaching a crisis point in

New Jersey, quite the opposite, in fact. My testicles looked like a pair of miniature armadillos curled up in their shells. A numb lump the size of a pinky finger had formed on my perineum, and my internal hemorrhoids felt like ground-up glass jammed up my butt.

At eighty-five miles, I hit a bump in the path and groaned demonstratively.

"Sorry about that," said Rivers, who had joined me at the midpoint of my ride and was supposed to warn me about such obstacles.

"It's okay," I said. "Just a beating for my two biggest haters."

"Your balls?" Rivers asked.

"No, not my balls," I said. "My hemorrhoids."

I explained to Rivers that I had named my hemorrhoids in honor of the two people who were working hardest to ruin my mission. One of them had created multiple fake Facebook accounts through which to slander me. The other had made a determined effort to prove I was committing charity fraud, not for justice's sake, but in the hope of seeing me disgraced and prosecuted.

Rivers laughed but stopped abruptly. "You're serious," he said.

"Now, whenever I hit a bump," I continued as though Rivers hadn't spoken, "it's not my body turning against me; it's me punishing my biggest haters."

I then stood on my pedals and executed a series of bunny hops, slamming my bike seat into my nether region at the apex of each jump.

"Take that!" I snarled. "And that! And that! And that!"

Psychologists call this type of behavior—putting a positive spin on negative events—cognitive reframing, and I was getting rather good at it.

As chance would have it, the turnaround point on our multi-lap bike course was the South Dakota State Penitentiary, an ugly brick complex that loomed off the left side of the path. Each time I came upon it I thought about the men inside and how happy many of them would be to trade places with me. *I don't have to ride my bike today*, I told myself. *I get to ride my bike today.*

Brian and his wife, Trish, had set up a staging area for me at the Sanford Sports Complex. After completing my bike ride (in seven hours and twenty minutes—one of my slowest times yet), I sat down on a patch of grass to eat before changing into running gear and starting the marathon. Rivers and Trish joined me on foot, and Lily and Lucy followed us on their bikes. We cruised along the same trail I had ridden on, facing the same wind, but I found it less bothersome at six mph than I had at 16. What did bother me was an odd tingling on the backs of my legs, which evolved into an itch, and then a burning, and then began to spread. Rivers noticed me fiddling with my shorts.

"Are you okay?" he asked.

"The whole back of my body itches like crazy," I said.

"Stop for a second," Rivers said.

I stopped. Rivers bent close to inspect my body.

"You've got hives all the way from your calves to your back," he said.

I pulled down my shorts.

"There too," he added.

Trish said I'd probably been attacked by chiggers, a species of mite, while sitting on the grass. We decided to head back to the staging area, where a tube of anti-itch cream was available inside the motor home. Rivers called Casey and Aaron to let them know we were coming. When we got there, we found the park swarming with young boys and their parents.

"Pee-wee football registration," Trish said.

The motorhome sat in the middle of the chaos. More conscious of time than of propriety, I positioned myself just inside the open door, facing in, and Rivers went to work rubbing cream into my legs and backside while Casey and Aaron stood guard on the steps. Attention focused on who knows what, the wingmen failed to notice a woman who came suddenly around the rear of the RV with her son in tow until it was too late to give warning.

"Excuse me," she said, addressing Casey. "Is this the sign-up for the junior football league?"

As these words hung in the air, the woman followed the wingmen's furtive glances toward the doorway, where Rivers could be seen crouching with both hands stuffed deep inside my shorts, rubbing my butt cheeks. Her jaw went slack.

"Yes, ma'am," Casey deadpanned.

More than 300 people showed up for the 5K, a new record—and in South Dakota, of all places, and for the first time, all five of my children participated. I couldn't help but notice that their legs were covered in the therapeutic tape I so often wore. My suspicion was that their participation and the taping were somehow connected, and it turned out I was right. Sunny informed me later that the kids had amused themselves after dinner by playing house. They were pretending to exercise and were all taped up. To them, this was life. People exercise, and when they need it, they get taped so that they can keep going.

During a break between the 5K and the last part of my marathon, one of my local supporters, Matt, tapped a Camel Lights cigarette out of its pack and lit it. I started running again before he'd finished the smoke. Instead of stabbing it out, Matt scrambled after me and sucked in the last few drags on the go.

"Can't say I've ever seen that before," I said to him.

"I'm trying to quit," he replied sheepishly.

Matt was not your typical triathlete. He smoked a pack and a half a day, worked as a carpenter, cursed like a sailor, and had brought three equally atypical buddies with him, one of whom sported a shaved head, two earrings, and a pair of nipple rings. They teased each other mercilessly, and I got the feeling they partied together as hard as they exercised.

"You'll quit when you're ready," I told Matt as he pocketed the butt of his cancer stick.

After that I said nothing more on the subject, knowing the best thing I could do to help Matt quit was shut up and run with him. The way I see it, all change is self-change. We can't make others do better. We can only empower them to *want* to do better. Indeed, although Matt and his friends had come out intending only to run the 5K, all four of them ended up running the last nineteen miles of the marathon— Matt's longest run ever—without any pressure from me.

As I glided into the night with my colorful companions, I remembered something that I had told a local radio reporter just that morning: "I'm not a person who will tell you what to do. I'd rather show you what is possible."

Shad and Dallas drove me to Bismarck in the van. When they slid open the door at sunrise on Day 46, I saw standing before me a handsome woman in her mid-sixties who wore white slacks and a blue-and-white-striped, short-sleeved top. My mother. I had known she was coming, but her sudden appearance at this early hour caught me off guard. I became acutely conscious of the IV catheter still stuck in my arm from the night before and of the locker room–meets–dog kennel stench surrounding me.

"Oh, Jay!" Mom said, erupting in tears.

My eyes welled too. Mom crawled right inside the van, and we held each other like refugees reunited after a long war.

"You've lost weight," she said, touching one of my gaunt cheeks.

"Not for lack of eating," I joked.

As if to underscore my point, Casey handed me my daily bowl of oatmeal. I gobbled it up and then strolled into the BSC Aquatic & Wellness Center with my expanded entourage. Mom, Sunny, and the kids huddled together in the poolside bleachers while I swam, easily visible from my lane.

Each morning I searched for one thing—some helpful thought or source of inspiration—to latch onto and get me through the pain of my swim. On this particular morning, I did not have to search.

I saw little more of my mother until evening when I delivered my pre-5K speech at Cottonwood Park. My North Dakota ambassador, Mark, had created a fine staging environment that featured a food truck, a sound system, tents, banners, an official race clock, and plenty of supporters. He had put his heart into this event, and he had pulled it off with bells and whistles. The atmosphere was tinged with awkwardness, for Mark was Jordan's father, and Jordan and I were five days away from possibly never speaking again.

Some friends are good for a laugh at a backyard barbecue. Other friends will have your back in a knife fight. I had known going into the campaign that Jordan was the first kind of friend, but I found out only during the coast-to-coast knife fight that was the Fifty that he wasn't the second kind. Jordan had been incredible before we started in Hawaii, but after we had begun, he had opted out of responsibility, and everyone else was working their butt off. Each time Jordan didn't do something he said he would do—whether it was making sure that merchandise orders were being fulfilled, or answering a sponsor request, or notifying an ambassador of a change in our plans, or simply having the van available at the staging area—another person had to step in. More often than not, that person was Sunny, who had become my de facto project manager while remaining the mother of five children who were constantly in her care, and the combined responsibility had taken a heavy toll on her.

Two days from now, Sunny would tell the video crew, "Emotionally, I feel like somebody shoved me into a pot and got a butter churn and went like this," making the motion of butter being churned, up and down with her arms.

I hoped I would be able to forgive Jordan eventually, but I would never forget.

By this point in our journey, my 5K speech was mostly rote, like a political candidate's stump speech. Among the many boilerplate sections that I repeated verbatim every day was this line: "I've got five kids: Lucy, Lily, Daisy, Dolly, and Quinn;

ages twelve, eleven, nine, seven, and five." When I spoke the last of these words in Bismarck, fifty members of my audience set off confetti poppers in perfect synchronization. For a moment I was stunned silent, but then I turned to Casey and Aaron and shook my head vengefully, fighting a smile.

"Apparently I need to change up my act a little," I said.

The dreamer and the sentimentalist in me comes from my mother. The athlete does not. She has always struggled with her weight, and she finds no joy in running. But as a gesture of support, and for her benefit, Mom had committed to run the last five Iron Cowboy 5Ks, preparing for the challenge by running intervals three times a week on a treadmill at her gym in Calgary. Having implored me not to allow her to hold me back, she jogged the first of these 5Ks at Cottonwood Park at her own pace while I trotted ahead. At the finish, I hung out and waited for her. And waited. And waited.

At last, long after everyone else had returned, I saw Mom laboring toward me from the park's edge, looking overwhelmed and embarrassed, but when she saw me, a smile of gratitude spread across her face. She came to me, and for the second time that day, we hugged like survivors.

In the early minutes of Day 47—that is, just after midnight—Mark's friend Lynn drove my mother and me to Bismarck Municipal Airport, where we squeezed inside a tiny four-seat plane that a friend of a friend had lined up for me. The nine-hour drive to Bozeman, Montana, which the rest of Team Iron Cowboy had embarked on long ago, would have been too long for me to make the start time for my next triathlon.

In the four hours we spent in the air, I slept maybe ninety minutes in short, shallow snatches. When I tried to sleep with my legs folded behind the pilot's seat, they cramped. When I stretched them out between the pilot's and copilot's seats, *they* fell asleep, waking me with the pins-and-needles pain of paresthesia. As we deplaned at Bozeman Yellowstone International Airport, I felt stiffer, more sore, and more dog-tired than at any moment of the Fifty.

Natalie, my massage therapist, whom I hadn't seen since Nevada, had driven up from Utah overnight. She fetched us from the airfield and delivered us to Bogert Park. Tim, my Montana ambassador, had provided a camper and parked it next to the Iron Cowboy RV. I stumbled in and passed out on the big bed in the back while Natalie worked on me. All too soon, a giggling mob comprising of Sunny, her friend Jenny, the wingmen, Shad, and Natalie burst into the motor home and turned my mattress into a trampoline. They were singing the lyrics to the DJ Snake and Lil Jon song "Turn Down for What," which blasted from Sunny's phone, as they jumped and rocked the camper. I pulled a blanket over my head.

When I got up, I found a Bozeman Barracudas swim cap on the kitchen table, left for me by Tim. I put it on and stepped outside and into a waiting crowd of boys and girls wearing the same swim cap. They went nuts.

Two hours later, I traded the latex topper for a bike helmet and rolled westward with a dozen others, including two guys named Greg, from Nashville, and Phillip, from Scottsdale. Two hulking guys, 6'4" musclemen, they went through the whole day with me. Greg rode a bike three sizes too small outfitted with old-fashioned toe cages. They wore unpadded running shorts and a flapping cotton T-shirt. The two of them winged it, not having any background in the sport at all. Greg and Phillip were like two overgrown Labrador retriever puppy, so boundless in energy and spirit that they were almost a danger to themselves, prone to dog-paddle too far from shore for the thrown stick. They had travelled together to come out and join me, showing their support and enthusiasm to anyone who crossed their path.

"Go big or go home!" they bellowed anytime someone asked if he was okay.

We pedaled all the way to the town of Three Forks, where the proprietors of the Sacajawea Hotel laid out a fabulous picnic lunch on white linen that made me feel I ought to change into something fancier before I sat down. We had just started back toward Bozeman when the Subaru crept past us with Shad at the wheel and Casey hanging halfway out the front passenger window. Strapped to the roof of the vehicle, as usual, was our kayak. Inside the kayak sat Aaron, paddling the air, his face dripping with water that Casey was squirting at him from a squeeze bottle.

"This urban kayaking in Montana is intense!" Aaron raved, serving as a play-by-play announcer to his own performance.

I lost it. My ribs shook so violently with the force of my laughter that my front wheel went squirrely and I had to quickly move my hands from the aero bars to the brake hoods to avoid going down. Ten minutes after Aaron had disappeared up the road, the absurd image came back to me and I nearly crashed again as I laughed out loud.

When we returned to Bogert Park, I found my father among the dozens waiting for me. He had just blown in from Calgary to make a brief appearance on his way to a BMW motorcycle owners club rally in Billings. We embraced stiffly and fell into embarrassed silence after trading breakfast-table banalities for thirty seconds. The two decades that had passed since I left home with my Ferris wheel contest winnings had not brought us any closer. Whenever I called home, and Dad answered, I said, "Hi, Dad," and he said, "I'll get your mother." He still wished I would get a real job and start being responsible. I still wished he would show me a bit of affection once in a while or offer some indication, any little sign, that he was proud of me and accepted me for who I am.

Knowing nothing of our quasi-estrangement, the video crew sat Dad down for an on-camera interview while I started my marathon.

"So what do you think of all this?" Jacob asked.

"I think it's crazy," Dad answered with a smile that was actually a frown at the corners. "It defies logic, what he's doing. He's doing good things, but it's not what I would choose to do."

Shocked by this lukewarm endorsement, Jacob gave him another chance.

"But it's for a great cause, right?" he prompted.

"I appreciate the cause," Dad said, eyes darting. "But I just wonder sometimes if he isn't preaching to the choir. The people he's attracting are already athletic."

Soon after these words were spoken, I ran the Iron Cowboy 5K with more than one hundred supporters. Among them was Gerry, a friend of Tim's who had been providing SAG support all day in Tim's pickup. Mostly sedentary and a little overweight, Gerry was so inspired by what he'd seen me do today that he made a spontaneous decision to jump into the 5K, his longest run ever. He finished ahead of only one person, and that was my father's wife, my mom.

⑱ CARNIVAL OF SWEAT

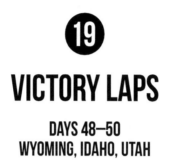

VICTORY LAPS

DAYS 48–50
WYOMING, IDAHO, UTAH

The first thing I saw when I walked inside the Jackson Aquatic Center was a big yellow corkscrew waterslide. I knew right away I would not be able to avoid giving it a try, and I put up little resistance when the wingmen marched me up the stairs and sent me whooshing down the slick plastic helix at the head of a human daisy chain.

I had encountered plenty of other waterslides during the campaign, and they hadn't tempted me in the slightest. But this was Day 48—I could almost see the finish line. The smoldering anxiety that I had carried around inside me for seven weeks had vanished overnight. When I woke up this morning and remembered my situation—forty-seven down, three to go—I relaxed deeply, as though exhaling a long-held breath. I felt like the leader of a long and grueling race who has just realized his chasers will not catch him and can begin to relish his triumph even before he crosses the finish line. Now certain of the Fifty's success, I looked ahead to these last three triathlons not as ordeals to survive but as rewards to savor. Victory laps.

My comeuppance came with about seven miles left in the marathon. I had just left the staging area at Jackson Hole High School with three companions for one last out-and-back on pitch-dark roads wet from earlier rain when I began to feel weighed down. A giant invisible thumb seemed to press my body into the pavement, which turned gluey, clinging to my shoes with every landing.

Time slowed to a syrupy ooze. We crept toward a stand of trees lining the left side of the road ahead with barely perceptible gradualness, trunks, and leaves frozen like a still life in the light of our headlamps. I checked my watch every five minutes

237

to find that only one minute had passed.

A bile surge of fear scorched my throat. This was not a bad patch; it was free-fall. My previous crises had been different in nature—crashes, cramps, panic attacks. Now I was just plain worn-out, fighting a losing battle against the same foe that stands between most triathletes and their goals in an iron-distance triathlon: good old-fashioned physical exhaustion.

"I've never hurt this bad before," I whispered to Kyle, who had rejoined the campaign that morning. "I don't know if I can make it."

"One step at a time," he said.

Kyle knew not to say too much, as did Jason, a Wyoming triathlete I knew from the racing circuit, who kept a respectful half step behind me, his face set in a frown of commiseration. My one other companion, Ryan, an ultrarunner from my native Calgary, did not. Ryan was a nice guy, and he meant well, but he talked too much and was helpful to a fault. He warned me about every puddle in my path and proposing earlier in the evening that he and others create a "man shield" to protect me from the wind and rain (not a bad idea, but did he have to call it that?).

As he prattled away, my fear transformed to anger, a generalized anger at everything but one that was sure to be unleashed on a specific target when it broke containment.

"How about we tell jokes?" Ryan asked.

"How about you shut up?" I snapped.

We came to a gentle rise in the road that might as well have been the stairs of the Empire State Building. My stride tightened up as though my legs had been lassoed. I reined back to a walk, balled my hands into fists, and howled in frustration. After a dozen steps, I continued running, as much to punish my body for its mutiny as to hasten the end of my misery.

Kyle suggested we shorten our current out-and-back, returning to the school for another break instead of trying to grind through the remaining miles in one shot as we'd originally planned. Back at the school, I grabbed a snack bar from the van, struggling to open the wrapper because I'd lost feeling in both ring fingers as a consequence of spending too much time with my forearms resting on my bike's time-trial bars, a position that pinched off circulation to the hands.

The only members of Team Iron Cowboy who hadn't left for Idaho Falls already were Sunny, Natalie, Carlee, and Jenny, who were sitting together inside Jenny's rental car catching up from being apart all summer. Natalie was also doing muscle work on a guy who had come out to support me. I tapped on a window, and it opened a crack. A warm draft wafted out. They were all laughing about something.

"Does anyone want to run with me?" I asked, sounding more pitiful than I'd intended to.

My words were met with a mix of mumbled apologies, and head shakes. Sunny was dressed in a skirt and flip-flops, so there was no way she could run with me. The window went back up.

We set out again at 10:58 p.m. Jason was not with us, having disappeared inside his truck and not yet reemerged. We'd gone no further than the edge of the parking lot when I heard footsteps behind me; Jason had rejoined the group wearing nothing but a black speedo with yellow smiley faces all over it. He had sported the same attire this morning at the pool, where he'd entertained me by performing underwater charades while I swam.

"What the heck are you doing?" I asked.

"You've got to finish the way you started!" he said.

I checked my watch: 22.83 miles. My brain was too tired to perform the simple arithmetic required to determine where I needed to turn around to return to the school at precisely the full marathon mark, so I delegated the responsibility to Ryan.

A marauding brain pirate was stomping through the corridors of my body's control room, randomly unplugging wires and disconnecting circuits. My field of vision—indeed, my entire conscious awareness—collapsed to a pinprick as I pressed ahead through ever-worsening depletion, yearning to hear Ryan's call for an 180.

Every few minutes, Kyle handed me a bottle. I would not have drunk otherwise. I splashed straight through the same puddles I'd carefully avoided on previous laps, no longer seeing them. My feet were soaked through and chafed raw. My knees felt arthritic. I pictured myself as an obese flamingo, legs ready to snap like Tinkertoys under my immense weight.

After twenty minutes that seemed like an hour, Ryan gave the word to reverse direction, and I told my body to stop moving. It obeyed. I then told my body to turn around. It did not obey, as if my feet were caught in rails—or might as well have been. My companions watched my static straining in puzzlement.

"A little help," I said.

Kyle and Ryan rushed to my sides and rotated me.

As I began the long homestretch to the night's finish line, I spoke to God. *Please have mercy on me,* I prayed. *I get the message: It's not over yet. Don't get ahead of your-*

self. Stay humble.

When my watch read 25.9 miles, we were still more than half a mile from the school. Ryan had botched the math. Apparently, God wasn't quite finished with my lesson.

"Ryan, do me a favor and go get the van," I said. "We'll wait for you."

Glad to have another shot at redemption, Ryan took off like a bullet. A minute later, Jason abruptly sprinted after him. When at last I hit 26.2 miles, I stopped dead in my tracks, bad idea. The blood abruptly drained from my head, and I wobbled. Kyle quickly grabbed hold of me. He was still holding me up when Ryan found us.

We drove back to the school to collect the girls. When we got there, I tried to climb out of the van to have a finish photo taken with Kyle, Ryan, and Jason, but it was beyond my current capabilities. I made it as far as the threshold before discovering that my legs just would not support me. So the others arranged themselves around me where I sat, Jason still wearing his speedo, and Natalie snapped a picture.

I then lay back on the van floor for the ride to Idaho Falls. For only the second time in the campaign, I did not shower after completing a triathlon; a man can't shower if he can't stand.

During the night I dreamed I was unable to start Day 49 because I couldn't find the pool.

"These are victory laps, man," I called out to Jacob as he filmed me on my bike from the window of a rented SUV in southeastern Idaho. "Two victory laps to go!"

How soon we forget. What can I say? God had taught me a lesson in Jackson. That lesson was instantly forgotten when I woke up in Idaho Falls feeling wholly revitalized, as though the previous night's catastrophe itself had been nothing more than a nightmare, and aware that the final finish line was that much closer. Yesterday I'd *thought* I was home free. Today I *knew* it.

Standing at the edge of the Idaho Falls Aquatic Center's indoor pool, I'd realized that, after this morning's swim, I would never have to swim 2.4 miles in a pool again if I didn't want to, and I didn't want to. Carlee jumped in with me and took the lead. Having been warned by Natalie, who had performed the same duty in Jackson, to expect slow going, Carlee was surprised when I began clicking off fifty-yard laps at a steady rate of one minute and forty-five seconds. This old horse was smelling the barn.

About a third of the way through my allotted distance we came to the wall to find Casey looming on the deck above us, gesturing for me to stop. With him was a woman who appeared to be about my mother's age, dressed to swim, looking bashful. I got the sense that she didn't swim often.

"This lovely lady would like to swim with you," Casey said.

"Just one lap," she said apologetically. "That's all I can do. I don't want to bother you, but it would mean a lot to me."

"Nothing would make me happier," I said with a welcoming smile.

Carlee took a lap off to allow this most unlikely supporter to paddle beside me, her age-stiffened arms making small strokes that did little more than stirring the water, her toothpick legs dragging behind unhelpfully. It took a lot longer than a minute and forty-five seconds to complete the trip, but I wasn't counting. We climbed out of the pool, took a quick photo, and then I got back to work.

When I looked for my new friend a few laps later, she was gone. I did not know how she had heard about me or what had inspired her to come here or why it meant so much to her to swim a single lap with me. I'm not sure I even got her name.

The bike ride was a party on wheels. A significant fraction of the twenty-plus cyclists surrounding me at any given time were friends from home, now just a half day's drive away. (My heart fluttered when we pedaled past a highway sign pointing the way to Salt Lake City.) The weather was what I would have ordered in every state if I could have: low eighties, bone dry, gentle breezes. In every photo I've seen from those six hours, I'm smiling.

The second-to-last Iron Cowboy 5K started at a local bike shop with another ample and vibrant group. When we came around the first bend in the course, I saw Casey and Aaron standing atop a rock formation in front of a small waterfall by the side of the road, costumed in grass skirts, coconut bras, and leis. I'd almost expected it.

Ryan, showing no hard feelings about my shushing him the night before, again ran the whole marathon.

"I can't believe you're doing this," he told me after nightfall, the group having thinned out to the usual core few. "When I saw you fall apart last night, I said to myself, *'He's done.' Nobody can come back from that kind of implosion and do an Ironman the next day.* How do you explain it?"

"There's something you don't know about me," I said.

"What's that?" Ryan asked, perhaps thinking he was about to hear some dark confession.

"I never have two bad days in a row."

We finished at 10:03, early enough that the motorhome had not gone ahead and my kids were still awake. A spontaneous celebration broke out. I embraced Aaron as though I had just completed Day 50, not Day 49. Lucy started up a chant of "U-tah! U-tah! U-tah!" and everyone else joined in, myself included, the girls kicking their legs up like cheerleaders, but then I noticed an absence, and my smile faded.

"Where's Sunny?" I asked.

Sunny was alone inside the motor home, prepping it for the night's drive, something she had spent ninety minutes a day doing for the past forty-nine days. Not long before I'd wrapped up my marathon, she'd had to interrupt the drudgery to referee a squabble between Lucy and Daisy. When that was settled, Lucy went outside to join everyone else. Dolly and Quinn were next, exhausted, they cried about who got to sleep where. As much fun as they'd had on this journey, these kids had been on the road for a long time. These awesome kids were exhausted, and they too were ready to get back to Utah.

As my question hung in the air, I spied Sunny's head through a small window on the side of the motorhome. She wasn't looking out at us in the hope of being noticed and pitied but was instead just quietly going about the necessary business. Caring for the kids on her own all summer, each night packing, folding and tidying the motorhome, taking care of the business side of the Fifty, and all of the things in between, all while everyone else was able to find time every day to do something fun. In Idaho, everyone was in earshot, chanting, cheering and celebrating as she continued working. My spirit sagged. The moment's symbolism was unambiguous. *This* was Sunny's Fifty.

The distinctive sound of tires rolling over a rumble strip scared me awake. Rivers had fallen asleep! The van was going off the road! It would roll over, and I would spend Day 50—*fifty!*—in an IC unit! The sound ceased and the van cruised smoothly onward.

"Are you okay?" I called out. "Do you need me to drive?"

Rivers and Sunny laughed at my anxiousness, at the absurdity of my taking the wheel now, of all times. Rivers explained that we were in a construction zone and had been traffic-coned into the breakdown lane. Nothing amiss.

Normally, Jordan and Jessa would have been the ones up front, but they had elected to make a stop at home in Salt Lake City before heading on to Provo for the big finish. I wasn't entirely sure they would bother to show up. I went back to sleep.

When I woke again, we were no longer moving, but it was still dark. When the van doors opened, there stood my friend Justin, who had been with me in Nevada, and someone in a giant, bunny costume. Everyone was laughing, but I was just confused, "Who is that?" I asked. Justin and Sunny laughed, they dragged out the prank for what seemed like forever. Finally, Sunny said, "Take off your head bunny!" When the head came off, it revealed the features of my old buddy Quinn from Calgary—the man I'd named my only son after. My heart nearly shot out of my chest. Quinn, Justin and I had spent several years as best friends, and it was a miracle that we were all there together, at the same time. I realized then that this was going to be the best day of my life—a wonderful and fearful thing to know.

Quinn grabbed the handle of the side door with a fluffy paw and flung it open. The scene behind him looked like a triathlon venue in the last predawn moments of race morning—cars, bikes, wetsuits, and fit-looking people everywhere. A local race director was even inflating buoys to place in the reservoir for my swim. I had been told to expect a sizeable turnout for my homecoming, and it appeared I would not be disappointed.

An informal receiving line formed at the side of the van. I reclined half awake, swaddled like a child king, and greeted one friend and supporter after another. Many of them were people I had met in previous states, fulfilling vows to make it to Utah if I did: Sarah from Texas, Lonnie from South Carolina, and Kevin from Massachusetts, among others. The last person to step forward was David, my teeth-grinding coach, whose life the campaign had probably shortened even more than my own. He smiled at me like a parent who has just gotten good news from the emergency room doctor.

"You look good," he said. "Some of those photos I saw from the past few days had me concerned. You seemed twenty years older."

At six thirty, Lucy and Lily sang the national anthem in front of the full gathering, eyes glistening. Already they were growing nostalgic for their summer of adventure, as was I.

The air at Deer Creek State Park (elevation 5,400 feet) was bracingly cold—in the upper forties—but I had been assured that the water temperature was close to seventy, so I chose my sleeveless wetsuit. The way into the water was rocky. I walked gingerly over the sharp edges on my shredded feet, Casey and Rivers each holding an elbow. Of the thirty-plus people creeping toward the reservoir, I must have appeared the least capable of completing an iron-distance triathlon.

The first step into the water felt like an unexpected slap to the cheek. It was frigid. Hadn't I promised myself in West Virginia that I would never again take anyone else's word on water temperature? I took a few more halting steps forward and then bit the bullet, immersing myself the rest of the way all at once. There were more heads than I could count bobbing in the water around me.

I began to swim. My supporters, having waited respectfully for this cue, followed suit, but they were so caught up in the energy of the moment that they took off as if the Ironman World Championship start cannon had just been fired. Face immersed, I felt the swimmers around me sprinting wildly, dragging and pushing me along. A blast of adrenaline sent my startled heart soaring to redline, dragging my lungs with it. I hadn't worn a wetsuit in several days, and I felt trapped inside it, starved for oxygen. Panic seized the wheel, and I began to hyperventilate. I couldn't feel my face, feet, or hands. Another swimmer clipped my foot, and I swallowed water.

When I stopped swimming, Casey and Rivers, ever vigilant, stopped with me. I lifted my goggles, revealing eyes like golf balls.

"I can't breathe!" I rasped.

Casey seized one arm and Rivers the other.

"Relax and float," Casey said. "We've got you."

When I was ready, I started to swim again. The panic had passed, but the farther I went, the colder I got. I stopped a second time.

"I can't do this," I said.

Casey and Rivers decided to take me to shore for a full reset, but would regret it. Although the sun had come up, the air was still much colder than the water. My teeth clacked between purple lips as I tried to put on a second wetsuit, donated by Shad. It took forever, and when the job was complete, the double layering only exacerbated the feeling of being buried alive, so I stripped down once again. At this point, there was nothing left to do but man up.

I waded back into the reservoir and gave it another shot. I had planned to swim 1.2 miles out, 1.2 miles in, but I turned around early in the insane hope that I would somehow cover more distance on the way back; of course, I did not. I finished what I sincerely hoped was the last swim I would do for a very long time by going back and forth in shallow water near my exit point, Casey checking my watch on my behalf at the end of each thirty-yard line.

As I was being helped out of the water, I told Aaron to hurry ahead and blast the heater in the van. When I got there a few minutes later, it was like a dry sauna inside. Casey, Aaron, and Sunny piled blankets on me and then smothered me in a pig pile for good measure. After twenty minutes of defrosting, I ventured to eat a plate of scrambled eggs. I was still trembling so badly that the food kept jumping off the fork, much to the amusement of my companions.

More than 150 supporters assembled on the park access road to ride their bikes with me. David gave a brief safety speech, instructing the others to stay behind me until we reached the bottom of the canyon, and then we launched. We turned right onto Route 189 and began a long descent toward Provo, tracing a route I had ridden countless times in training—indeed, the very route of which I had dreamed up the idea for my first world record attempt. The majestic Wasatch mountains jutted brutally skyward on either side of us, all limestone and dolomite, looking every day of their 300 million years.

We bottomed out at the junction of Route 52 and swarmed into civilization. As we approached the Riverwoods shopping center, my face went slack. Another 250 cyclists awaited me in the parking lot, like a cavalry receiving their general. The vision jarred me almost outside myself. Suddenly I was twenty-three years old again, fresh off the Ferris wheel, and by some strange magic, I was here, granted a vision of where it would all lead. I turned to Casey and Aaron, both of whom intended to go the full distance with me today.

"I'm just James," I said inanely. "I'm just James."

The two pelotons merged and flooded into Provo, pouring down University Avenue like a tidal wave, swallowing cars and people in an unstoppable flow. We emerged out the south side of the city and began to arc around Utah Lake, stringing out over several miles as I held a tempo up front that most couldn't match. A three-wheeled roadster, driven by Justin and Quinn, still in a bunny suit, pulled up alongside us. Why not? Soon after that, a police cruiser with lights flashing and sirens blaring raced past us and pulled over in the bike lane ahead. An officer leaped out and commanded us to stop. The symmetry of the moment was uncanny. Twenty miles into Day 1, I was pulled over by a cop. With twenty miles to go on Day 50 . . .

IRON COWBOY

"Don't stop," my friend Shane told me. "I'll handle this."

That was good enough for me. I kept going. I don't know what Shane said to the lawman, but we didn't see him again.

The ride ended at Electric Park, at Thanksgiving Point, in the town of Lehi. Arriving there was like walking into a surprise birthday party times fifty. Everyone I knew was present, plus hundreds of people I didn't know, all pressed between tents, booths, and food trucks that offered everything from triathlon club memberships to smoothies. If I had parachuted into the midst of it all unawares, I would have assumed I had landed at some kind of fitness festival. (Actually, now that I think about it, parachuting in would have been really cool!)

After a short trip to the weathered motorhome for food and a change of clothes, I started the marathon with more than forty supporters, most of them pledging to cover the entire distance. When I'd completed the first mile, my watch beeped. I looked at the time. 9:58. *I need to slow down,* I thought.

I couldn't slow down.

After an hour and a half of running in the ninety-degree heat, many in the group had run out of fluids and were suffering, so we looped back to the park, arriving there at fourteen miles. The crowd had swelled enormously. More than 3,500 people had decided they would rather witness and/or participate in the completion of my journey than do anything else they might have done on this beautiful Saturday in late July.

It was getting on toward six o'clock when I headed back out. A quick bit of mental arithmetic informed me that if I hustled, I could somehow manage to cover nine miles in the next seventy minutes. I would then be left with just 3.1 miles, to complete the Fifty, when the Iron Cowboy 5K started at seven. For once, as originally intended, my finish line could be everyone's finish line.

I began to run brisk one-mile loops around and through the two-square-block park, now as densely packed with spectators as the concert grounds at an outdoor rock festival. David and Rivers flanked me, brushing aside the many supporters reaching out with Iron Cowboy postcards and pens.

"What's my pace?" I asked Dave.

"It's 7:53 per mile," he said.

I sped up. When we thundered down the path that cut through the middle of the park, the huge crowd exploded, pressing close on both sides. I took it up another notch, impelled by an energy that was not entirely physical, feeling no tiredness

246

whatsoever, no sense of limitation. The runners behind me fell away like debris from a disintegrating rocket. More than a few decided they'd had enough and quit. My pace dropped to 7:35 per mile, then 7:17, and lower still.

Each time I came back around, the multitude erupted anew, unleashing a celebratory roar that boxed my ears and left them ringing. Again time slowed, but welcomely now. My senses were animal sharp; I heard every voice, saw every face, some of them familiar, most of them not. There were male faces, female faces, young faces, old faces, white faces, brown faces, thin faces, round faces, all of them open-mouthed and hollering, celebrating this bizarre and wonderful thing we'd created together.

My last big push paid off. At seven o'clock, always the official but seldom the actual start time of the Iron Cowboy 5K, I was exactly 5K away from completing my mission. About half of my supporters now changed roles, going from spectators to partakers, and filed out behind me. I was no longer in any rush. Mincing along at the slowest pace that qualified as running, I stopped for hugs, selfies, autographs, bathroom breaks, and refreshments. After fifty days of wanting to finish, to be done with it all, I now wanted this crazy ride to go on forever.

Also, I was afraid of tomorrow. What was I going to do when I woke up in the morning and realized there was no lake to swim, no road to ride, no trail to run? What would take the place of the do-or-die purposefulness of my life in the last fifty days? What kind of void would I face when my beloved tribe dispersed?

At twenty-six miles, I signaled to Tyrell, the man responsible for my first triathlon in a cowboy hat, and he announced my final approach over the PA system. I made one final turn and then came down the homestretch between rows of flags representing all fifty states, low-fiving supporters with both hands, Lucy beside me, Rivers and Dallas behind me, Casey and Aaron stoking the crowd ahead of me, confetti flying above me, cameras everywhere. It was all so incredibly real, and yet at the same time dreamlike. I was wholly inside what was happening but somehow also outside it, thinking, *I can't believe this is happening.* Four steps away, three steps...

My whole life flashed before my eyes. No, seriously. I saw it all: the referee raising my ruined left arm after my last wrestling match, the disappointment in the eyes of my Paris mission president when I told him I wanted to go home, the Ferris wheel, the wheelchair at the fights, my wedding day, the repo man, David's frozen smile when I dropped the Fifty on him, my lower legs swollen to the bursting point on Day 7 in Flagstaff, Arizona, a desolate street in suburban Wichita at three o'clock a.m. on Day 11, Sunny's face when I woke up in wet cycling shorts with a bottle of

IRON COWBOY

kombucha in my hand on the RV's foldout bed on Day 17 in Henderson, Kentucky, Mom finishing her fourth consecutive last-place finish in last night's Iron Cowboy 5K in Boise. Each image stood in precise alignment with the others on a vector that ended right here, right now. In the blink of an eye, the vision passed, leaving behind an overpowering sensation of letting go, of release, completion.

Two steps . . . I saw Sunny, Lily, Daisy, Dolly, and Quinn's faces behind the finish arch. I felt my face erupt in a stupid grin. And then, at 8:05:39 p.m. on July 25, 2015, with one final step, a journey of 96,980 swim strokes, 1,265,537 pedal revolutions, and 2,579,038 running strides (not to mention 12,610 miles of vehicular and air travel)—a journey that wasn't about numbers at all- ended.

⑲ VICTORY LAPS

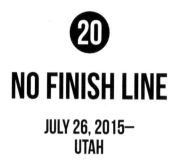

NO FINISH LINE

JULY 26, 2015–
UTAH

The guys from *Success* magazine arrived at our new rental home in Orem at eight o'clock on a gloomy Wednesday morning in the middle of September. After a brief exchange of handshakes and pleasantries, I showed them into the living room, where I sat down with Jesus, the writer, for a lengthy interview about the Fifty, then seven weeks behind me, while Derek, the photographer, snapped candids and his assistant, John, held a light screen.

"The thing with the Fifty was that there was only one person who needed to believe in me, and that was myself," I told Jesus near the end of our conversation. "To anyone who is trying to accomplish a big goal, I would say the most important thing is to have 100 percent conviction in what you're doing."

When the interview wrapped up, we moved out to the garage. I had agreed to lead Jesus through a strength workout while Derek took more photos.

"Let's get a few with your shirt off," Derek said. "The art director specifically requested abs shots."

"I'm not taking my shirt off," I said flatly.

"Why not?" Derek asked.

"Because I'm fat. I've gained twenty pounds."

"Oh, come on!" Derek said. "You look great. Let's see them. Lift up your shirt."

I lifted up my shirt—very briefly.

"I would kill for that stomach," Derek said.

"The shirt stays on."

My downward spiral began on the very night the Fifty ended. The celebration at Electric Park lasted until almost midnight. Sunny and the kids and I then made our way to our friend Liz's house, where we'd camped out for the last six weeks before the Fifty. We still had no place of our own. It was close to 1 am when I finally laid down to sleep, sleep that I'd looked forward to for a very long time.

An hour later, I woke up screaming. Both legs were electrocuting themselves with muscle spasms. Sunny massaged one leg while I rubbed out the other.

"Why is this happening now?" I asked.

Eight O'clock the next morning, a team from Rudy Project, my eyewear sponsor, came by to do a photo shoot. One look in the bathroom mirror told me how ill-conceived that idea had been. I looked like a man who'd spent the last fifty days lost in a jungle. I went through with the shoot, but the images were unusable.

Media requests poured in all day long. CNN wanted to talk to me. FOX News called. Everyone insisted on studio interviews in Salt Lake City—a forty-five-minute drive each way. The interviews themselves would last just three minutes apiece, and yet I felt obligated to accept every invitation. This was my big chance to parlay the Fifty into new opportunities, but my head was filled with fog, and all I really wanted to do was go back to bed.

The fog persisted in the following days. Meanwhile, other symptoms emerged—like bloating. I had body scans done on the first and third days after the campaign's conclusion, and I ballooned from 5.0 to 7.7 percent body fat in that short span of time. Every major joint in my body ached, and I couldn't decide if this was something new or if my brain was only now allowing me to perceive it. I avoided staircases as much as possible. Going down hurt especially, producing a bone-on-bone grinding feeling in my knees. One week after the Fifty, I was far less capable of completing an iron-distance triathlon than I had been at any point during it.

The thought of exercising made me shudder. I figured this was natural enough, but as the days turned into weeks, my motivation to work out remained at an all-time low. When the crew from *Success* came to see me, I still hadn't run a single step since the Fifty. I was obliged to admit this to Jesus when, after we'd completed our garage workout, he suggested we go for a short run on the scenic Bonneville Shoreline Trail near my home. Assuming I was sandbagging, Jesus did the same, assuring me I couldn't possibly be in worse shape than him. It took all the pride I could muster to hide my pain under a poker face as we jogged back and forth in front of Derek's lens.

Exacerbating my physical decline was the failure of my appetite to adjust to my sudden sedentariness. The constant hunger I had experienced throughout the campaign continued for some time afterward. I craved all of the wrong foods, and I had no ability whatsoever to resist my cravings. The confluence of inactivity and overeating wrought predictable results. I gained twenty-eight pounds in three months.

As my chiseled physique disappeared under a thickening layer of blubber, I began to struggle with my identity. Was I still the Iron Cowboy? Would people not take me seriously if I showed up for speaking engagements looking like a middle-aged accountant? Would they lose all interest in me if I didn't follow up the Fifty with other feats of endurance? And what did I want for myself—to hold on or move on?

I finally hit bottom on August 18. That night I lay awake in bed next to a sleeping Sunny brooding on the Fifty and its aftermath. My thoughts on this subject—and it was the only subject I thought about—came in two flavors: grievance and regret. I tried to shut off the negative chatter, but I couldn't find the switch. Eventually, I gave up and padded into the kitchen to fix myself a snack I did not need. As I sat at the table and ate, I played around distractedly with my phone. Before I knew it, I was working my thumbs feverishly, typing out a rambling soul dump on a guy I'd hired to help me write a book. I barely knew him, yet I held nothing back.

I'm awake and can't sleep. I'm upset, and I don't know why. It's been a month since I finished and I'm still in a huge funk and incredibly confused about my role, my expectations. I remember very little about the summer and people keep asking me how I did it. I don't know how I did it. I woke up. I swam. I rode. I ran. I just did it. That's what you do when you start something—you do it, you finish it. I don't know how to articulate what happened. Few will ever understand how great a feat this was. What I did and how I did it. What I overcame. I had to go somewhere else to do this, somewhere I can't explain, and now it's all a waste. I ruined Sunny's summer. No, Jordan did, and that's my fault. I wanted this to be spectacular. I wanted it to be perfect. I failed at raising money. People accuse me of self-promotion. Am I a fraud? How do you shout from the rooftops "look at me" to try to raise funds and at the same time not self-promote? I can't do one without the other. People accuse me of doing this for myself. Maybe I am a selfish jerk, and I did do this for myself, to prove to everyone I'm a bad-A. But who am I really? I had so many long conversations with myself out there on the road, how could I possibly not know? Everyone wants my advice, my opinion, but doesn't want to pay me for it. How do I feed my family if I give everything away? How do I remain humble and at the same time want to be recognized for doing what was impossible? I'm lost and going to bed.

My physical and emotional states were unimproved a month later when I spoke at an event hosted at Communal, an upscale restaurant in Provo. My audience was a bunch of millionaires—attendees of an invitation-only conference for executives and entrepreneurs in the tech industry. I have a great fear of public speaking. Before each event, I freak out and come up with some lame excuse to cancel. Only my sense of shame stops me. My anxiety is most extreme when I know I'm going to be out of my element—and at Communal I knew that I would be way out of my element.

My friend Sid, who organized the event, introduced me. As I stood in the wings listening to him talk me up (did these people even know what an Ironman was?), I felt an overpowering urge to regurgitate my breakfast. *Just be yourself,* I said inwardly. *Just tell your story.* And that's what I did. It's what I always do because it's the only thing I know how to do. More than twenty years after my ill-fated mission in Paris, I'm still the world's worst evangelist—still not one to preach or pitch.

Anyone who has stood up in front of people as many times as I have, knows it doesn't take long to sense whether one is bombing or killing it. Ten minutes after I stood up in front of the millionaires, I realized—to my astonishment—that I was killing it. All eyes were fixed unwaveringly on my face. Some of my expensively suited listeners were perched well forward in their seats. Occasionally, one of them whispered into the ear of another, who then nodded. They laughed at all the right places.

Any doubt I might have had about how my story had gone over was snuffed out during the question-and-answer session. Every person in the room raised a hand at one time or another. Some asked about me—about my diet, perhaps, or methods of time management. Others shared something about themselves and asked for advice, but all seemed able to personalize my journey in some way—to identify with it and take something away from it. The fact that what I had done was inconceivable was not an impediment to these connections, but the very key to them. The sheer extremity of the Fifty made it universal. The challenge that had been hard enough to push me to the breaking point symbolized the big challenge that each person was facing in his or her own life.

Later that same week I spoke before a very different group at Sharon Elementary School in Orem, where Casey had taught until the end of the preceding school year. As the father of a gaggle of grade school children, I had a good sense of how to tweak my presentation to make it understandable and exciting to my young audience. Instead of describing an Ironman in terms of miles or meters, I told the students that I rode my bike from our present location to the Idaho border every day. That blew their minds. I made sure to show them a photograph of the disgusting toe blister that caused me such grief in Missouri. They squealed and shaded their eyes and writhed in their seats, loving it.

Overall, though, I told pretty much the same story I had told the millionaires. And I got the same reaction. The kids watched me with that saucer-eyed, slack-mouthed look my younger ones take on when I read a favorite bedtime story, and they were as full of questions as the wealthy guys and gals, although, as you can imagine, the nature of the questions was quite different. ("Were you, like, super smelly the whole time?")

I drove home tingling with excitement. At last, the fog had lifted. I saw the way forward now, and the way forward was no different from the way I had come. To find my footing in my life after the Fifty, I realized, all I needed to do was be myself and do what felt right, as I always had. At Communal and again at Sharon Elementary School I had touched people—two very different groups of people—simply by sharing my story. Doing this had felt almost as natural to me as doing the Fifty itself, and its impact was similar as well. In both situations, people came out to glimpse an average guy who had dared the impossible and went home believing they could do their own impossible.

How many people could I touch in this way?

Looking to raise my game as a public speaker, I hired a professional speaking coach. He sat in on a couple of my events and offered feedback and guidance on how to improve my act. I did everything he asked me to do: traded my casual clothes for a suit, shaved my beard, and added pithy take-home lessons to my slideshow. "Just be yourself," Sunny kept saying, but I felt like I needed to make sure that I was "good enough" to be speaking, doing it the way "they" do it. The first thing I noticed after I'd made all these changes was that I wasn't having fun anymore. (Although I dreaded every event, I actually enjoyed almost all of them once I had the microphone—until I started trying to be someone I wasn't.) The next thing I noticed was that my audiences didn't seem as engaged or as deeply affected as they had before.

Lessons don't empower, living examples do. Before I hired my public speaking coach, when I just stood up in front of people and told my story, everyone could relate to it in one way or another. My journey met each person where he or she was. Lessons bled the life out of the living example of the Fifty, and not just the life but also the truth. My speaking coach wanted me to tell people that achieving goals and dreams was a simple five-step process, or nine-step process, or whatever. Well, it isn't. Completing a journey takes as many steps as there are steps in the journey, and you don't get to the end by applying lessons. You get there by making the decision to take each step until there are no steps left to take. To do that, you need nothing more than the belief that you can. Such a belief comes mostly from within, but it can be fed by the examples of others—like me.

I eventually shared these concerns with Sunny and Tyrell and asked for their advice. They told me to fire my speaking coach, so I did. I then hung the suit up in the closet, got rid of the lessons, and yes, I even regrew the beard.

Around the same time I made the mistake of hiring a speaking coach, I was contacted by a Hollywood casting director, Sami, who was recruiting talent for a new reality TV show, which he described as "*Ninja Warrior* meets *Survivor*." He said he thought that I would be perfect for the show. I couldn't have agreed more. I let Sami know I was in, and the vetting process began. First, I filled out an online application. Then, I did a Skype interview. After that, I underwent a psychological examination, also via Skype. To my amazement, I passed the psych test and was invited to take the final step: a "callback" in Los Angeles. When I saw the date, my heart sank. I sent Sami the following email:

I have put a lot of thought into this, and unfortunately, I am going to have to withdraw from the casting process. It kills me to do this because I want the spot. I was made for a show like this. I am the toughest, most mentally strong person you'll ever meet. What I lack in physical strength, I more than makeup for with my mind. I proved it this past summer. Holy crap, I did fifty Ironmans in a row through fifty states! Not one person thought I could do it, but I did.

I would be free on the 29th of October, but it just happens to be my eldest daughter's birthday (she is turning thirteen) and I promised her that I would be home. I simply cannot break this promise to her.

I do hope you understand and will consider me for future opportunities with your casting company.

Respectfully,
James Lawrence
The Iron Cowboy

Part of knowing who you are, and what kind of person you want to be, is knowing who you aren't, and what kind of person you don't want to be.

As I traveled throughout The United States and the world sharing my story and empowering employees, students, servicemen and servicewomen, and athletes, other good things began to happen. My hunger for training and competition gradually returned, and I began the long process of transforming my body and rebuilding my fitness. The first time I got back in the pool, I was surprised to discover that I actually enjoyed swimming again. My delight was tempered somewhat, however, by the equally surprising discovery that my much-abused right shoulder still hadn't healed entirely. Over the next several months, with Dallas's and Natalie's help, it returned to 100 percent. Okay, 95 percent.

My first big post-Fifty competition was a two-day team relay triathlon in Utah called Dóxa, whose organizers had designated it "the official race of the Iron Cowboy." My team included Casey, Aaron, and Rivers, all of whom showed up fitter than they'd been during the Fifty, when their own training had been forced to take a backseat. We won by two and a half hours. (Sunny, Dallas, Brittany, and Carlee competed as well, on another team.)

Dóxa is not a USA Triathlon–sanctioned race, so Casey and I could have done it even if we had been banned by the United States Anti-Doping Agency (USADA) for receiving saline IVs before participating in the HITS New York Triathlon on Day 36. Fortunately, we weren't banned. David filed our self-reporting paperwork the day the Fifty ended. After a long and tedious process (much of it during the Fifty), when at some points the outcome did not look promising, we were cleared of any wrongdoing. Not only that, but USADA agreed to alter the language of the rule we had unwittingly broken so that in the future only athletes who receive a saline IV before a sanctioned race for the purpose of gaining a competitive advantage are penalized.

I wish I could say that I've achieved my goal of raising $1 million to combat childhood obesity, but I also still believe I will before it's all said and done. It will just take more time than I had originally intended. In the meantime, I continue to support various charity efforts. As I write these words, I am planning on mountain biking to the top of Mt. Kilimanjaro in March of 2017, with two other guys, in an effort to raise $1.9 million for Treasures for Africa Home for Children. Like I said before, sometimes the good you do is not the good you expected to do.

Other loose ends left dangling after the Fifty were also tied up once I had my mojo back. My father and I started communicating. Somehow we came up with a "question-a-day" routine in which we took turns asking each other anything, be it trivial or pointed or in between, through the Voxer app. (It's huge in Canada.) The game petered out after a while, but not before it had thawed the chill that had existed between us for so many years and helped me understand him better, and vice versa.

One night, while the question-a-day thing was still ongoing, a friend reached out to me through Facebook and directed me to a vicious personal attack that had just been levied against me on the social media website. Its author was a guy named Nick, someone I knew already as one of my biggest haters. In fact, he was the very agitator who had started the Elliptigate controversy.

I decided to send Nick a private message. Resisting the temptation to call him a jerk and challenge him to a fight, I instead merely defended myself against the specific accusations he'd made and asked him why he hated me so much. In turn, there was a heated back-and-forth exchange through which it emerged that Nick admitted that he was simply jealous. An accomplished ultra-endurance athlete himself, Nick envied my Fifty experience and the recognition it brought me. He wanted me to fail and to fall into disgrace because my success made *him* feel like a failure, reminding him that the only reason he hadn't attempted something like the Fifty himself was that he lacked the courage.

Attacking a person on social media out of jealousy is not the same as being a jerk. To his credit, Nick came around, eventually reciprocating my reasonable and respectful (though firm) manner of communicating with him. I feel confident saying that he is now an Iron Cowboy fan and that our dialogue helped him to accept a very different and far less negative picture of who I am. I am more than the guy that he had imagined to suit his purposes.

On June 6, 2016, exactly one year after the Fifty kicked off at the YMCA of Kauai, Sunny launched a public Facebook diary in which she shared her own memories of the journey. Writing under the title *Tri the Other Side,* she covered one state each day for fifty days with characteristic candor. Reading these chronicles was painful for me, even shaming at times. I knew Sunny had suffered along the way but not how much, or specifically, how, because she never told me. The stress and strain of the Fifty had traumatized her so deeply that she couldn't bear to revisit it. As the anniversary approached, Sunny's instincts told her that sharing her side of the story, not only with me but with the public, would be therapeutic, and it was. In her final entry, she wrote, "Don't buy into the idea that we live in a world of sadness, hurt, and evil. During this journey, we experienced far more love and generosity . . . than we [did] bad or hard experiences."

I'm still a dreamer, and I always will be. My dreams have evolved, focusing on, strengthening others and helping them also to believe in their personal ambitions and goals.

In March 2016, David and I launched Team Iron Cowboy, an online community for triathletes and runners. Aaron and Carlee are among our coaches. We're open to everyone, but our membership skews toward the beginner end of the experience spectrum. Our mission is to bring the magical, transformative experience of crossing finish lines to as many people as possible. Endurance sports aren't for everyone—there are other worthy goals to pursue—but I have found that people often achieve those other goals in the very process of chasing finish lines. Somehow it has a way of instilling in people the belief and the never-quit attitude that are needed to achieve goals of all kinds.

I also dream of reaching as many individuals as I can with the Fifty. To this end,

I continue to speak around the world, I released the video documentary that Jacob and his boys at Mystery Box created for me, and I wrote this book. The Fifty itself may have ended, but through these vehicles, it inspires and empowers people no less effectively now than it did in my direct interactions with the men, women, and kids who came out to swim, bike, and run with me between Hawaii and Utah.

Truth be told, I am also keeping the Fifty alive for my own sake. One of the questions I heard most often during the campaign was "What's next?" I hated this question for what it implied. Nobody asked Neil Armstrong what was next while he was still on the moon! I thought it should be as obvious to others as it was to me that the Fifty was a culmination. *Nothing* came next; no other challenge of its kind could ever follow it. I mean, what would it be? Swim, bike, and run around the equator? Complete nine iron-distance triathlons in nine days, one on each planet of the solar system?

"I've played my Man Card," I said time and again to those who posed the "What's next?" question, "and I'm not putting it back in the deck."

I understand that people who are wired to explore limits often have a hard time knowing when to quit, but I guess I'm different. While I hope always to be an athlete and to pursue physical challenges, I do not feel eternally compelled to top myself, to get just one more fix of the going further drug. I do miss the Fifty, though, and knowing that I will never experience anything like it again makes me miss it all the more.

We did more living in those fifty days, my team and I, than some people do in as many years. I feel the most aching nostalgia when I sift through my memories, see particular photographs, or bump into someone I associate with that singular experience. A part of me yearns to go back, to be there again, in that indescribably special pocket of time when my kids were a certain age, when Sunny and the wingmen and I were bonded like soldiers, and I was at the height of my strength and the limit of my endurance, and the end was not yet known.

ACKNOWLEDGMENTS

Where do I even begin? So many people have helped me in so many ways on the journey that has brought me here. I had no clue how hard—or how fulfilling—writing a book could be, and I'm sure glad I didn't have to do it alone.

I owe a similar debt of gratitude to the fifty-plus ambassadors and the countless other volunteers who supported my team and me as we swam, biked, ran, drove, and flew our way across America (and back) in the summer of 2015. Without their generosity, my dream to *Redefine Impossible* would not only have been impossible to achieve, but also meaningless. It was the shared struggle, the camaraderie, and teamwork, that made it worthwhile. I should add that this tip of the cowboy hat also goes out to the many friends, associates, and strangers who helped me in the pursuit of my two Guinness World Records and all the way back to the beginning of my endurance quest.

It wasn't only the people who labored on my behalf who gave my journey significance. No less important were the men, women, and children who participated in it by swimming, cycling, or running with me, or just by showing up to see me, or by following it remotely. The Iron Cowboy Army helped me succeed by wanting me to succeed, and I hope they got back as much as they gave.

Having read this far, you know how important a role my various sponsors played in enabling me to go after my goals and empower others. I treasure each of these relationships, from the greatest to the smallest, but I wish to give special acknowledgment to Gary and Mary Young. They have been my most abiding supporters, sharing both my passion and vision for doing the impossible. Much love and gratitude to Vaughn Cook of ZYTO, Chris Washburn at Fezzari, Rene Oehlerking at Jaybird, Paul Craig and Devin Johnson at Rudy Project, and Jeremy Howlett at Altra.

The bonds I forged with the official and more-or-less-official members of the team that surrounded me during the Fifty are so special to me that just thinking about them brings tears to my eyes. Thank you, Dano Dayton, Tyrell Gray, Dallas Makin, Tommy 'Rivers' Puzey, Natalie Rasmussen, Carlee Tulett, Kyle Woodruff, Brittany Light, and Garen Winn.

My loyal wingmen have been left off this list because their unique sacrifices and contributions deserve a shout-out of their own.

Thank you, Aaron Hopkinson for keeping the mood calm, always having my equipment ready, and for giving me your summer. Your focus was always on the Fifty and on me. You drove so many nights, without any relief, and always managed to stay cool and calm. Thank you!

Thank you, Casey Robles. Every minute, of every day, you kept us all smiling and managed to turn hard moments into moments of fun and resolution. Your driving will forever be remembered, as will your dancing, but your loyalty to my family and me is what I will remember most. Leaving your family for the summer was a tremendous sacrifice, and you stepped right in and helped Sunny to care for mine while I wasn't able. Thank you!

To my coach David Warden, my loyal friend and the mastermind who put together my training for the Fifty, I could not have done this without you! You are honest and possess an integrity that is rare and valuable. It is an honor to have you share your brilliant mind with me, getting me through my accomplishments. It is even a greater honor to have you working as the head coach for Team Iron Cowboy. Thank you will never be enough, and I am forever indebted to you.

I am grateful and indebted to my family for reasons that go way beyond this book and my athletic undertakings, but are also inseparable from them. I thank my father-in-law and mother-in-law, Ron and Maurine Hatfield, for their unconditional support and for always believing in me. My parents, Alan and Charlotte Lawrence, raised me right and taught me so many valuable lessons. I have done well in this world, and it is because of what my parents taught me.

Finally, I offer my deepest thanks to my wife and soul mate, Sunny Jo, for loving and accepting me as I am, yet also inspiring and motivating me to be better. There is no other woman in this world for me. You are the sunshine I see in the morning, and the stars I see when I lay down at night. Thank you for being my best friend, companion, and the mother of our beautiful children.

Thank you to my kids, Lucy, Lily, Daisy, Dolly, and Quinn. Each personality adds to the bounty of our home. Lucy, thank you for your dedication, determination, and sarcasm. You have always supported me and been excited about each adventure. Lily, thank you for your smiles, magic, and sparkles that you spread everywhere that you go. Your red hair and freckles are as special as you are in our family. Daisy, thank you for sharing your warm heart. Your hugs, smiles, and gentility are precious, and I look forward to them every day. Dolly, thank you for being you, which is absolutely one-of-a-kind. Thank you for your unique fashion, your confidence, and your deep and genuine love for life and people. Quinn, thank you for your enthusiasm and joy for life. With every jump, prank, and smile you give, you remind me that life is full of energy and can be fun no matter what the circumstance may be.